MRCOG Part 1

400 SBAs
Second Edition

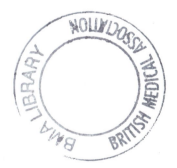

MRCOG Part 1

400 SBAs
Second Edition

Katherine Andersen MBBS BSc MRCOG
Specialty Trainee in Obstetrics and Gynaecology
North Middlesex University Hospital NHS Trust, London, UK

Tara Woodward MBBS BSc (Hons) DRCOG PgDip Journalism
General Practice Trainee
North Middlesex University Hospital NHS Trust, London, UK

William Dooley MBBS BSc MMed
Specialty Trainee in Obstetrics and Gynaecology
Imperial College Healthcare NHS Trust, London, UK

Edited by
Maryam Parisaei MRCOG
Consultant Obstetrician and Gynaecologist,
Homerton University Hospital NHS Foundation Trust, London, UK

Amit Shah MRCOG
Consultant in Reproductive Medicine and Surgery,
Homerton University Hospital NHS Foundation Trust, London, UK

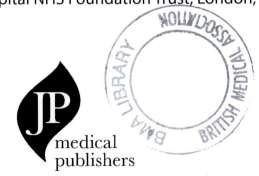

JP
medical
publishers

London • Philadelphia • Panama City • New Delhi

© 2016 JP Medical Ltd.
Published by JP Medical Ltd
83 Victoria Street, London, SW1H 0HW, UK
Tel: +44 (0)20 3170 8910   Fax: +44 (0)20 3008 6180
Email: info@jpmedpub.com   Web: www.jpmedpub.com

ISBN: 978-1-909836-46-4

British Library Cataloguing in Publication Data
A catalogue record for this book is available from the British Library

Library of Congress Cataloging in Publication Data
A catalog record for this book is available from the Library of Congress

Commissioning Editor:	Steffan Clements
Editorial Assistant:	Adam Rajah
Design:	Designers Collective Ltd

Foreword

The Membership of the Royal College of Obstetricians and Gynaecologists (MRCOG) remains the cornerstone for the assessment of knowledge required by trainee doctors in the UK. Passing the exam is a prerequisite for progression through the structured training programme towards the Certificate of Completion of Training (CCT) and entry on to the Specialist Register. The standard of the exam remains high and the curriculum is based on UK practice.

The MRCOG Part 1 exam can be taken at any time after graduation but it must be passed before the transition from ST2 to ST3 of the training programme. This book aims to provide an exam revision guide for trainee doctors in ST1 and ST2, and international candidates preparing to sit the exam.

For international graduates often working outside of recognised training programmes, it is a tough exam to pass. Despite this, many international graduates continue to take the exam knowing that success will demonstrate the acquisition of knowledge to a high standard, which will enhance the treatment of the women and babies in their care.

The MRCOG Part 1 has changed in the last few years. It has always tested the knowledge base in all the basic sciences as they pertain to obstetrics and gynaecology, but the examination now contains only single best answers (SBAs). This allows the syllabus to be tested in a more clinically relevant manner. Doctors planning to take the exam must know how to answer the SBA format, and for this they require exam technique and clinical knowledge.

In this second edition there are 400 SBAs – 25% more than in the first – which have been updated to account for changes in practice and guidelines. Covering all the core sciences as well as current RCOG clinical recommended practice, *MRCOG Part 1: 400 SBAs, Second Edition* provides a comprehensive revision aid with helpful explanations after each question. At the back of the book there are two practice papers for readers to test their knowledge and practise exam technique.

Maggie Blott FRCOG
Consultant in Obstetrics and Maternal Medicine,
Corniche Hospital Abu Dhabi
Former Vice President (Education) of the
Royal College of Obstetricians and Gynaecologists, UK
May 2016

Preface

We are delighted to present *MRCOG Part 1: 400 SBAs, Second Edition*. The format of the questions used in the exam has changed since the publication of the first edition to consist solely of single best answers (SBAs). This revised second edition reflects the new format.

This book covers the breadth of the MRCOG Part 1 syllabus, allowing the candidate to work through all subject areas before attempting full length versions of Paper 1 and 2 under timed conditions. Within the answer sections, references are made to the latest evidence-based practice, and tables and diagrams are used to aid in the assimilation of this information.

The philosophy of the book remains the same; by practicing questions in a systematic manner, candidates will build their confidence and be able to approach the exam knowing they have covered the syllabus. Passing the MRCOG Part 1 remains a major achievement, but we believe that with appropriate preparation, success at the first sitting is achievable.

Katherine Andersen
Tara Woodward
William Dooley
Maryam Parisaei
Amit Shah
May 2016

Exam revision advice

Exam format

The MRCOG Part 1 exam is composed of Paper 1 and Paper 2. Each paper consists of 100 single best answer (SBA) questions and is equally weighted with 50% of the marks available for each. Each paper must be completed within two hours and thirty minutes (150 minutes).

Single best answer (SBA) questions

SBAs comprise of three components: a stem (most commonly a clinically relevant vignette), a lead in question and five answer options. The answer options are homogenous and are presented in alphabetical or numerical order for ease of reference.

Candidates should read the question carefully then select the single most appropriate answer from the five options.

The nature of a SBA means that there are four distractors surrounding the correct answer. Of the four distractors, there may be one or two distractors which can reasonably be identified as incorrect. There are also likely to be one or two distractors that are plausible answers. At this point candidates will need to read the stem and lead in question again, then make a judgement as to which answer fits best.

How to use this book

We believe that one of the best ways to revise for the exam, and crucial to passing at the first attempt, is to work through practice questions again and again. In this way, confidence will be gained with the new question format and the full curriculum will be covered.

We have included two mock exam papers at the end of the book, which can be completed under timed conditions to provide a good sense of the time constraints of the real exam. Allow two and a half hours to sit each paper.

Finally, having a study buddy is a good way to maximise exam preparation. In addition to keeping each other on track, you will be able to help with areas of the curriculum that your buddy may be struggling with. We studied for the exam together, which gave us focus, a timetable to keep to and some friendly competitiveness to make sure we took our exam preparation seriously.

Tara Woodward
Katherine Andersen

Contents

Chapter 1

Anatomy

Questions

For each question, select the single best answer from the five options listed.

1. An 82-year-old woman attends her general practitioner's surgery complaining of a painful lump in the groin.

    Which of the following does not form a boundary of the femoral triangle?

    A   Adductor longus
    B   Inguinal ligament
    C   Obturator internus
    D   Pectineus
    E   Sartorius

2. A 32-year-old woman complains of pain in the right buttock. She is 36 weeks pregnant and has a history of chronic back pain.

    Which nerve supplies the gluteus maximus muscle?

    A   Inferior gluteal
    B   Internal obturator
    C   Internal obturator (lateral cutaneous nerve of the thigh)
    D   Sciatic
    E   Superior gluteal

3. Following a routine elective caesarean section, the rectus sheath is being sutured.

    With regards to the rectus sheath, which of the following is correct?

    A   Arcuate line demarcates the upper limit of the posterior layer of rectus sheath
    B   External oblique aponeurosis forms the posterior aspect of the sheath
    C   Internal oblique aponeurosis always passes in front of the rectus abdominis
    D   Scarpa's fascia is superficial to Camper's fascia and the external oblique
    E   Transversalis fascia lies directly below the rectus sheath

4. A 47-year-old woman undergoes a routine transabdominal hysterectomy to remove a large fibroid uterus. She is found to have a fibroid in the broad ligament, and there is concern that her ureter may have been damaged during the operation.

    With regards to the path of the ureter, which of the following is correct?

    A   In the broad ligament, both ureters pass over their respective uterine artery
    B   It runs lateral to the internal iliac artery

     C Ovarian vessels enter the pelvis posterior to the ureters
     D The upper third of the ureters lie in the abdomen
     E Ureters cross close to the bifurcation of the common iliac vessels

5. What structure does the right ovarian vein empty into?

     A Azygos vein
     B Inferior vena cava
     C Internal iliac vein
     D Right renal vein
     E Right pudendal vein

6. A 27-year-old woman has a forceps delivery under regional anaesthetic. She suffers multiple second degree tears to the lateral vaginal wall.

Sensory innervation of the vagina is provided by which nerve?

     A Dorsal nerve of the clitoris
     B Inferior hypogastric plexus
     C Inferior rectal nerve
     D Obturator nerve
     E Pudendal nerve

7. Which artery supplies the structures derived from the foregut of the embryo?

     A Coeliac trunk
     B Inferior mesenteric
     C Middle rectal
     D Renal
     E Superior mesenteric

8. A 73-year-old woman undergoes a laparoscopic-assisted vaginal hysterectomy and oophorectomy. There is a large bleed during the procedure, so it is converted to a laparotomy.

Which of the following provides the arterial blood supply of the left ovary?

     A Abdominal aorta
     B External iliac artery
     C Internal iliac artery
     D Left ovarian artery
     E Obturator artery

9. During a laparoscopic-assisted vaginal hysterectomy, the surgeon accidentally damages the ovarian artery.

With regards to the left ovarian artery, which of the following is correct?

     A It anastomoses with the vaginal artery
     B It is a branch of the abdominal aorta
     C It follows the course of the left ovarian artery

    D It lies inferiorly to the inferior mesenteric artery
    E It supplies both left and right ovaries

10. Which of the following arteries is a terminal branch (not paired) of the abdominal aorta?

    A Gonadal
    B Median sacral
    C Phrenic
    D Renal
    E Suprarenal

11. Following a forceps delivery, a 32-year-old woman has an episiotomy repaired.

    Which of the following does not insert into the perineal body?

    A Bulbocavernosus
    B External anal sphincter
    C Ischiocavernosus
    D Levator ani
    E Transverse perineal

12. Following a failed trial of instrumental delivery, a woman undergoes an emergency caesarean section at full dilatation. A lateral extension to the uterine excision is bleeding.

    Which of the following gives the correct pairing of artery and its origin?

	Artery	**Origin**
A	Internal pudendal	Posterior division of internal iliac
B	Ovarian artery	Common Iliac
C	Testicular artery	Abdominal aorta
D	Uterine artery	Abdominal aorta
E	Uterine artery	Anterior division of the internal iliac

13. Which of the following is not part of the bony pelvis?

    A Fourth lumbar vertebrae
    B Ilium
    C Ischium
    D Pubis
    E Sacrum

14. Which of the following describes the anatomy of the inguinal region?

    A The deep inguinal ring lies at the lateral two-thirds of the inguinal ligament
    B The deep inguinal ring transmits the ilioinguinal nerve
    C The superficial inguinal ring lies below the pubic tubercle
    D The superficial inguinal ring transmits the genitofemoral nerve
    E The superficial inguinal ring transmits the round ligament

15. Which of the following nerves is transmitted by the superficial inguinal ring?

    A Femoral nerve
    B Genitofemoral nerve
    C Ilioinguinal nerve
    D Peroneal nerve
    E Sciatic nerve

16. A 24-year-old primiparous woman has been in second stage of labour for 90 minutes. There is a bradycardia, so a decision is made for a forceps delivery. She does not have an epidural, so she is given a pudendal anaesthetic. Upon examination, the presenting part is in a direct occipito anterior position at the +2 station.

    With regards to the pudendal nerve, which of the following is most accurate?

    A It arises from the posterior rami of S2, S3 and S4
    B It supplies the piriformis muscle
    C It leaves the pelvis through the lesser sciatic foramen
    D It supplies the clitoris
    E It crosses over the ischial tuberosity, lateral to the internal pudendal artery

17. A 28-year-old woman suffers a 4ᵗʰ degree tear following a water birth. This is repaired in theatre. The medical student on attachment on the Labour Ward asks you about the anatomy of the anal canal.

    Which of the following statements would you choose to describe the anal canal?

    A The upper half is lined with cuboidal epithelium
    B The lower half is lined with keratinised stratified squamous epithelium
    C The fibres of ischiococcygeus form part of the internal anal sphincter
    D The dentate line lies at the border of the upper one-third and lower two-thirds of the anal canal
    E Hilton's line indicates the junction between keratinised and non-keratinised stratified squamous epithelium

18. A 42-year-old woman is undergoing her fourth caesarean section on the elective list at 39 weeks' gestation. The procedure is complicated by dense adhesions of the anterior abdominal wall.

    Which of the following statements most accurately describes the rectus sheath?

    A The rectus sheath is made up of the aponeuroses of transversus abdominis and internal oblique
    B Below the arcuate line, the posterior rectus abdominis is separated from the peritoneum by transversalis fascia and connective tissue
    C Pyramidalis is external to the rectus sheath
    D The rectus sheath contains the ventral rami of lower eight thoracic nerves
    E Contains an anastomosis between the internal thoracic artery and superior epigastric artery

19. Superiorly, the vagina:

A Receives its arterial blood supply from the uterine arteries
B Receives its lymphatic drainage via the inguinal lymph nodes
C Receives its venous supply from the ovarian vein
D Receives somatic innervation via the pudendal nerve
E Is lined with secretory columnar epithelium

20. A woman is taking oral steroids daily as part of treatment for an acute flare of inflammatory bowel disease. She is admitted to labour ward at 37 weeks' gestation in active labour and is commenced on IV steroids as there is concern about adrenal insufficiency.

The adrenal glands can best be described by which of the following?

A The left adrenal gland is triangular-shaped
B The adrenal cortex consists of chromaffin cells
C The right adrenal vein drains into the right renal vein
D Part of their nerve supply is provided by the thoracic splanchnic nerves
E The left adrenal gland is in contact with the descending colon

21. A 28-year-old primiparous woman is taken to the operating theatre for a trial of instrumental delivery as she has been pushing for 90 minutes and the presenting part has reached the ischial spines station. She is Caucasian and her height is 152 cm. The baby seems to be of a normal size, but you are concerned about the adequacy of the pelvis.

Which is the most accurate description of the diameters of the pelvis?

A The anatomical anteroposterior diameter (true conjugate) is approximately 11 cm
B The obstetric conjugate is larger than the true conjugate
C The anatomical transverse diameter forms the largest pelvic diameter (approximately 15 cm)
D The antero posterior diameter bisects the true conjugate
E The coccyx forms an important bony landmark in measurement of the pelvic outlet

22. A 38-year-old woman undergoes a diagnostic laparoscopy for chronic pelvic pain. She is suspected to have pelvic venous congestion.

Which is the best description of the veins of the pelvis?

A The left ovarian vein drains directly into the inferior vena cava
B The external pudendal vein passes through the pudendal canal
C The uterine venous plexus lies medially to the broad ligament
D The internal pudendal vein drains into the great saphenous vein
E The rectal venous plexus is a site of portocaval anastomosis

23. During a difficult second stage caesarean section for failure to progress, there is a right uterine angle tear. You suspect that the right ureter may have been injured whilst applying haemostatic sutures.

The ureters are muscular tubular structures and:

    A   Lie in front of the peritoneum
    B   Are 35 cm long
    C   Cross in front of the uterine arteries
    D   Originate embryonically from the ureteric buds
    E   Insert into the bladder posteromedially

Answers

1. C Obturator internus

The femoral triangle is an anatomical area in the upper thigh. The borders of the femoral triangle can be remembered by the mnemonic SAIL:

- Sartorius (laterally)
- Adductor longus (medially)
- Inguinal
- Ligament (superiorly)

The floor of the femoral triangle is formed by the iliopsoas laterally and pectineus medially. Important structures passing through the femoral triangle include the femoral nerve, artery and vein (**Figure 1.1**).

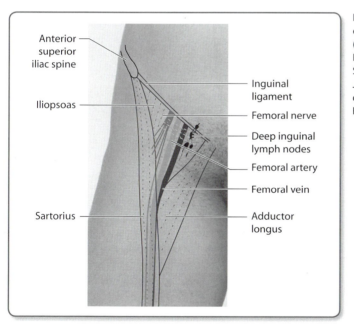

Figure 1.1 Anatomy of the femoral triangle. (Reproduced from Tunstall R and Shah N. Pocket Tutor Surface Anatomy. London: JP Medical Ltd, 2012 and courtesy of Sam Scott-Hunter, London.)

Anterior superior iliac spine

Iliopsoas

Sartorius

Inguinal ligament

Femoral nerve

Deep inguinal lymph nodes

Femoral artery

Femoral vein

Adductor longus

2. A Inferior gluteal

Gluteus maximus:

- Origin: posterior gluteal line of inner upper ilium, posterior surface of lower sacrum, lumbodorsal fascia and sacrotuberous ligament
- Insertion: iliotibial band, ischial tuberosity
- Nerve: inferior gluteal
- Artery: superior and inferior gluteal arteries
- Action: extension and external rotation of hip

3. E Transversalis fascia lies directly below the rectus sheath

The rectus sheath is formed from the aponeuroses of three muscles: transversus abdominis, external and internal oblique muscles. Above the arcuate line, the aponeurosis of the external oblique passes in front of the rectus abdominis and the transversus abdominis passes behind; the aponeurosis of the internal oblique divides into two at the lateral margin, with the anterior lamellae passing in front of the rectus abdominis and the posterior lamellae passing behind. Scarpa's fascia is deep to the Camper's fascia and superficial to external oblique muscle. See **Figure 1.2** for the anatomy of the rectus sheath above and below the arcuate line. The transversalis fascia forms the layer below the rectus sheath.

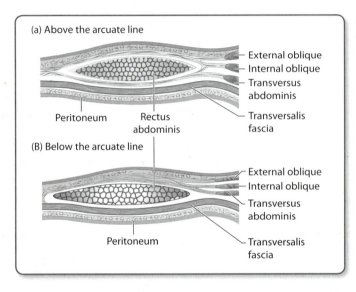

Figure 1.2 Anatomy of the rectus sheath.

4. E Ureters cross close to the bifurcation of the common iliac vessels

The ureters leave the kidney and travel inferiorly and medially along the psoas muscle. They run along the posterior pelvic brim and cross anteriorly to the bifurcation of the common iliac vessels. They continue posteroinferiorly and turn medially at the ischial spines. They then run in the base of the broad ligament where they are crossed by the uterine artery ('water under the bridge'). The ureter passes the lateral vaginal fornix and enters the bladder.

5. B Inferior vena cava

The right ovarian vein empties directly into the inferior vena cava. The left ovarian vein empties into the left renal vein before reaching the inferior vena cava.

6. E Pudendal nerve

The pudendal nerve provides sensory innervation to the vagina. The pudendal nerve passes into the urogenital region at the end of its course and gives rise to the perineal branches, which supply the vagina and posterior two-thirds of the vulva. It also gives rise to the dorsal nerve, which supplies the clitoris.

7. A Coeliac trunk

The embryonic foregut forms the mouth to the duodenum. The coeliac trunk is the first branch of the aorta once it has passed through the diaphragm. The coeliac trunk then branches into three: to the left gastric artery, the splenic artery and the common hepatic arteries. The superior mesenteric artery provides blood supply to the embryonic midgut and the inferior mesenteric to the embryonic hindgut.

8. D Left ovarian artery

Both ovaries receive their arterial supply from the ovarian arteries, which are direct branches of the abdominal aorta. Venous drainage of the right ovary is supplied by the right ovarian vein, a branch of the inferior vena cava (IVC). Venous supply of the left ovary is from the left renal vein, which then drains into the IVC. The differing blood supply of the ovaries, in comparison to the other pelvic viscera, reflects the embryonic origin and subsequent descent of the ovaries from near the kidneys, down into the pelvis.

9. B It is a branch of the abdominal aorta

The ovarian arteries arise from the abdominal aorta. The paired blood vessels, which sit below the renal arteries and above the inferior mesenteric artery, descend along the posterior abdominal wall and cross the external iliac vessels at the level of the pelvic brim. Each artery supplies its respective ovary and fallopian tube, anastomosing with the uterine arteries. Arterial and venous supply to the ovaries follow a similar course, but the right ovary receives its venous supply from the right ovarian vein, which reaches the inferior vena cava, and the left ovary is supplied by the left renal vein.

10. B Median sacral

The aorta enters the abdomen through the aortic hiatus of the diaphragm at the level of T12. At the level of L4, the abdominal aorta bifurcates into the common iliac vessels, which in turn divide to form the external and iliac vessels. The abdominal aorta has three terminal branches, which are right and left common iliac arteries and the median sacral artery. There are another four paired branches, which are phrenic, suprarenal, renal and gonadal arteries.

11. C Ischiocavernosus

The perineal body (or central tendon of the perineum) is a midline structure formed of fibromuscular tissue found between the vagina and the anus in females. The external anal sphincter, transverse perineal muscles, bulbocavernosus muscle and the levator ani muscles all insert into the perineal body. The ischiocavernosus muscle lies in the superficial pouch of the perineum. Lying between the perineal membrane and the subcutaneous tissue, it arises from the inferior ischial ramus and compresses the crus clitoris, hence promoting clitoral erection. See **Figure 1.3** for the anatomy of the perineum.

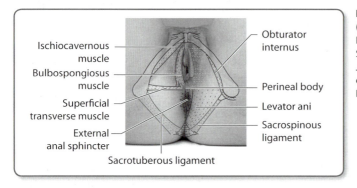

Ischiocavernous muscle
Bulbospongiosus muscle
Superficial transverse muscle
External anal sphincter
Sacrotuberous ligament
Obturator internus
Perineal body
Levator ani
Sacrospinous ligament

Figure 1.3 Perineal body. (Reproduced from Tunstall R and Shah N. Pocket Tutor Surface Anatomy. London: JP Medical Ltd, 2012 and courtesy of Sam Scott-Hunter, London.)

12. E Uterine artery, Anterior division of the internal iliac

The uterine artery is a branch of the anterior division of internal iliac artery (the main artery to supply the pelvic viscera). Ovarian arterial supply comes from the ovary arteries which are direct branches of the abdominal arteries. Equivalent to the female ovarian arteries is the testicular artery, which is a branch of the abdominal aorta and supplies the testes. The internal pudendal artery, which supplies the perineum, is a branch of the anterior division of the internal iliac artery.

13. A Fourth lumbar vertebrae

The bony pelvis consists of the innominate bone, which is formed from the ilium, the ischium, the pubis, the sacrum and the fifth lumbar vertebrae. The sacrum itself is formed from the five sacral vertebrae, and articulates with the fifth lumbar vertebrae. **Figure 1.4** shows the structure of the bony pelvis.

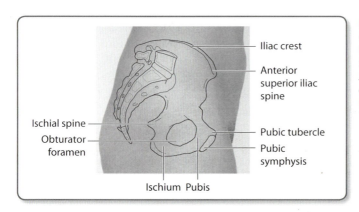

Ischial spine
Obturator foramen
Ischium Pubis
Iliac crest
Anterior superior iliac spine
Pubic tubercle
Pubic symphysis

Figure 1.4 Bony pelvis. (Reproduced from Tunstall R and Shah N. Pocket Tutor Surface Anatomy. London: JP Medical Ltd, 2012 and courtesy of Sam Scott-Hunter, London.)

14. E The superficial inguinal ring transmits the round ligament

The deep inguinal ring is situated at the midpoint of the inguinal ligament. It can be located by finding the midpoint between the anterior superior iliac spine and the pubic tubercle. The superficial inguinal ring lies just above, and lateral to the pubic tubercle. The deep and superficial rings mark the entrance (deep ring) and exit (superficial ring) to the inguinal canal.

The canal's boundaries are:

- Anterior wall: external oblique aponeurosis, with lateral reinforcement from the internal oblique
- Posterior wall: transversalis fascia, with the conjoint tendon (internal oblique and transversus abdominis) providing medially
- Superiorly: internal oblique
- Inferiorly: inguinal ligament

Running through the canal is the round ligament in females and the spermatic cord in males. The ilioinguinal nerve passes through the superficial inguinal ring only, having travelled down the lateral abdominal wall between the internal and external oblique muscles. See **Figure 1.5** for the anatomy of the inguinal canal.

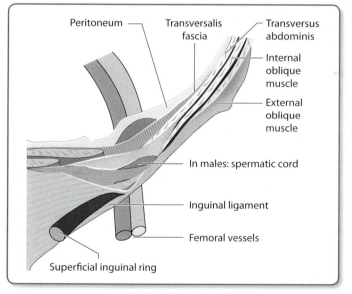

Figure 1.5 Anatomy of inguinal canal.

15. C Ilioinguinal nerve

Only the ilioinguinal nerve passes through the superficial inguinal ring; it is not carried through the deep inguinal ring, having travelled down the lateral abdominal wall between the internal and external oblique muscles.

16. D It supplies the clitoris

The pudendal nerve originates from the anterior (ventral) rami of S2, S3 and S4. After passing between piriformis and coccygeus, it leaves the pelvis through the greater sciatic foramen. It then crosses the ischial spine with the internal pudendal artery and re-enters the pelvis through the lesser sciatic foramen. The pudendal nerve passes medially to the internal pudendal artery (**Figure 1.6**).

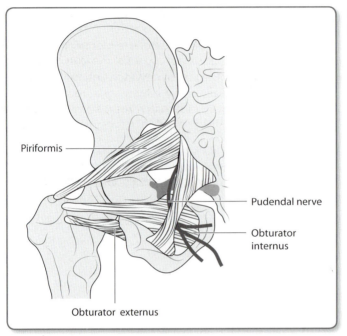

Figure 1.6 Anatomy of the pudendal nerve.

Piriformis

Pudendal nerve

Obturator internus

Obturator externus

17. E Hilton's line indicates the junction between keratinised and non-keratinised stratified squamous epithelium

The anal canal is approximately 3 cm long and lies between the anorectal junction and the anal orifice. The upper two-thirds are lined with cuboidal epithelium and are supplied by the superior rectal artery. The lower third is lined with non-keratinised stratified squamous epithelium and is supplied by the inferior rectal artery. At the anal orifice there is a transition to keratinised stratified squamous epithelium with the presence of sweat glands and hair. Hilton's line is a white line which indicates the junction of the keratinised from the non-keratinised epithelium. The pectinate line is an important embryological landmark which lies at the junction of the upper two-thirds and lower one-third. The fibres of pubococcygeus blend with the internal anal sphincter.

18. B Below the arcuate line, the posterior rectus abdominis is separated from the peritoneum by transversalis fascia and connective tissue

The rectus sheath is formed from the aponeurosis of the transversus abdominis, internal and external oblique muscles. At the lateral margin of the rectus abdominis, the internal oblique splits into an anterior and posterior layer, passing in front and behind. In front of the rectus abdominis runs the external oblique aponeurosis and the anterior layer of internal oblique. Behind the rectus runs the posterior layer of internal oblique and the transversus abdominis. The aponeuroses of each side meet at the central linea alba. Below the arcuate line, all aponeuroses pass in front of the rectus abdominis, meaning that the posterior aspect of the lower third of rectus is separated from the peritoneum by transversalis fascia and extraperitoneal connective tissue. The ventral rami of the lower seven thoracic nerves and anastomosis between the superior and inferior epigastric vessels occurs within the rectus sheath. Where pyramidalis is present, it lies within the rectus sheath anterior to rectus abdominis.

19. A Receives its arterial blood supply from the uterine arteries

In outline, the blood and nerve supply to the vagina are:

- Artery: superior – uterine artery
        inferior – vaginal artery
- Vein: vaginal vein
- Lymph: superior – internal iliac nodes
        inferior – superficial inguinal nodes
- Nerve: sympathetic – lumbar splanchnic plexus
        parasympathetic – pelvic splanchnic nerves

20. D Part of their nerve supply is provided by the thoracic splanchnic nerves

The adrenals (or suprarenal glands) sit below the diaphragm and above the kidneys. The left gland has a semi-lunar shape and sits proximal to the spleen, pancreas and stomach. The right triangular adrenal gland sits slightly lower than its counterpart, making contact with the liver and inferior vena cava (IVC). The outer cortex of the glands originates from mesoderm and is responsible for corticosteroid and androgen production. The inner medulla derives from neural crest cells and its chromaffin cells secrete catecholamines. The glands receive their blood supply from the suprarenal arteries (superior, middle and inferior). The left suprarenal vein drains into the left renal vein and the right suprarenal vein drains into the IVC.

21. A The anatomical anteroposterior diameter (true conjugate) is approximately 11 cm

The diameters of the pelvis can be broadly categorised into transverse, anteroposterior and oblique (**Figure 1.7**). The anatomical transverse diameter is approximately 13 cm. It is the obstetric transverse diameter that bisects the true conjugate.

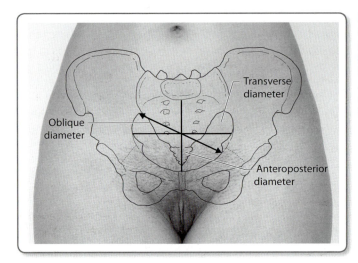

Figure 1.7 Anterior view of the female bony pelvis. (Reproduced from Tunstall R and Shah N. Pocket Tutor Surface Anatomy. London: JP Medical Ltd, 2012 and courtesy of Sam Scott-Hunter, London.)

22. E The rectal venous plexus is a site of portocaval anastomosis

The right ovarian vein drains directly into the inferior vena cava. The left ovarian vein drains into the left renal vein. The internal pudendal vein drains into the internal iliac vein and the external pudendal vein drains into the great saphenous vein. The internal pudendal vein passes through the pudendal canal with the pudendal artery and nerve. The uterine plexuses lie in the superior angles of the uterus, between the two layers of the broad ligament. They connect the ovarian and vaginal plexuses and drain directly into the hypogastric vein. The two other sites of portocaval anastomosis are in the oesophagus and hepatic circulation.

23. D Originate embryonically from the ureteric buds

Ureters are muscular tubular structures approximately 25 cm long, which run along the posterior abdominal wall. They are retroperitoneal through their entire course and carry urine from the kidneys to the bladder. The ureter begins at the kidney and descends from the renal pelvis along the medial border of the psoas muscle. From there, it enters the pelvis and crosses the common iliac artery. In females, the ureters travel in the broad ligament and run under the uterine artery before inserting into the bladder posterolaterally.

Chapter 2

Biochemistry

Questions

For each question, select the single best answer from the five options listed.

1. Which condition is caused by the failure to mineralise newly formed osteoid?

   A Osteomalacia
   B Osteopaenia
   C Osteopetrosis
   D Osteoporosis
   E Paget's disease of bone

2. Six weeks after sustaining a distal radial fracture, a 50-year-old woman presents to her general practitioner complaining of fatigue and upper abdominal pain. Her blood tests indicate hypercalcaemia and hypophosphataemia.

   What is the most likely diagnosis?

   A Bone metastases
   B Increased parathyroid hormone-related protein production
   C Primary hyperparathyroidism
   D Sarcoidosis
   E Secondary hyperparathyroidism

3. Which enzyme is involved in the rate-limiting step of the glycolysis pathway?

   A Glucokinase
   B Glucose 6-phosphate
   C Hexokinase
   D Phosphofructokinase
   E Phosphoglucose isomerase

4. What is the overall product of the glycolysis pathway?

   A Glucose
   B Pyruvate
   C 1 NADH + 1 ATP
   D 2 NADH + 2 ATP
   E 4 NADH + 4 ATP

5. A 28-year-old primiparous woman attends her booking appointment at 10 weeks' gestation. She is keen to maintain a healthy diet during her pregnancy and asks her midwife to explain the difference between essential and non-essential amino acids.

Which of the following is a non-essential amino acid?

A   Arginine
B   Leucine
C   Methionine
D   Tryptophan
E   Tyrosine

6. A 24-year-old woman is admitted via the emergency department with persistent hyperemesis of pregnancy. She is now feeling very unwell and appears dehydrated. Her blood pressure is 110/60 mmHg, her heart rate is 100 beats per minute, her blood oxygen saturation level is SpO_2 98% on room air and she has a respiratory rate of 20 breaths per minute.

Which is the most likely acid-base disorder in this patient?

A   Metabolic acidosis
B   Metabolic alkalosis
C   Mixed metabolic alkalosis and respiratory acidosis
D   Respiratory acidosis
E   Respiratory alkalosis

7. Following the birth of their second child with severe developmental delay, a couple is seen by a clinical geneticist. Genotyping suggests a rare autosomal recessive condition caused by a defect in the normal functioning of the citric acid cycle.

Which of the following is not an intermediate of the citric acid cycle?

A   Alpha-ketoglutarate
B   Acetyl coenzyme A
C   Citrate
D   Oxaloacetate
E   Succinyl coenzyme A

8. Which of the following describes the appearance of sister chromatids during the anaphase of mitosis?

A   Alignment along the cell's horizontal plane
B   Alignment along the cell's vertical plane
C   Alignment at one pole
D   Separation to diagonal poles
E   Separation to opposite poles

9. A 12-year-old boy has gross developmental delay of unknown cause. On physical examination, he is noted to have macro-orchidism, prominent ears and a large forehead. He is seen by a clinical geneticist who suspects Fragile X syndrome and wishes to perform genotyping.

    Which of the following laboratory techniques is used to detect DNA sequences?

    A   Eastern blotting
    B   Northern blotting
    C   Northwestern blotting
    D   Southern blotting
    E   Western blotting

10. A 58-year-old woman has recently been diagnosed with type 2 diabetes mellitus. As part of her routine care, her general practitioner checks her fasting cholesterol levels. She is found to have a mildly raised total cholesterol level with a raised serum low-density lipoprotein level.

    Which of the following describes the function of low-density lipoproteins?

    A   Transport of cholesterol from the body's tissues to the liver
    B   Transport of cholesterol from the liver to tissues around the body
    C   Transport of chylomicrons from the liver to elsewhere in the body
    D   Transport of triglycerides from the intestine to other tissues for storage
    E   Transport of triglycerides from the liver to elsewhere in the body for oxidation

11. An infant is born at term by normal vaginal delivery. When the baby is 18 days old, his parents bring him to the emergency department. He is vomiting, severely dehydrated and appears to be underweight. The paediatricians diagnose a salt-wasting crisis and are concerned that he has a form of congenital adrenal hyperplasia.

    What hormone deficiency is characteristic of this disorder?

    A   Cholesterol
    B   Cortisol
    C   Dihydrotestosterone
    D   Oestradiol
    E   Testosterone

Answers

1. A Osteomalacia

Pregnancy is associated with increased levels of parathyroid hormone, calcitriol and calcium. Higher concentrations of calcium are absorbed from the gut. Calcium and phosphate are transferred to fetal circulation by active transport.

See **Table 2.1** for conditions associated with abnormalities of bone.

Table 2.1 Disorders of the bone and their typical serum biochemistry					
Condition	Calcium	Phosphate	Alkaline phosphatase	Parathyroid hormone	Comment
Osteoporosis	Normal	Normal	Normal	Normal	Decreased bone mass
Osteopetrosis	Normal	Normal	Normal	Normal	Marble bone disease
Osteomalacia Rickets	Reduced	Reduced	Increased	Increased	Soft bones
Osteitis fibrosa cystica	Increased	Reduced	Increased	Increased	Brown tumour
Paget's disease of bone	Normal	Normal	Increased	Normal	Abnormal architecture of bone

2. C Primary hyperparathyroidism

Parathyroid hormone (PTH) leads to an increase in blood calcium and a reduction in phosphate. Primary hyperparathyroidism causes hypercalcaemia by increased secretion of parathyroid hormone, in 80% of cases from an adenoma of the parathyroid gland. Other causes include hyperplasia or multiple adenomas. It is the third most common endocrine condition, with a population frequency of 1:500–1:1000. Symptoms are usually those of hypercalcaemia. Blood tests usually show increased calcium and PTH and low phosphate. Treatment involves surgical removal of the adenoma. Secondary hyperparathyroidism consists of high PTH, but low calcium. Bone metastases would lead to hypercalcaemia, but not hypophosphataemia.

3. D Phosphofructokinase

Glycolysis is the metabolic process that produces two molecules of pyruvate from one molecule of glucose. This process of glucose oxidation also generates a gain of two molecules of ATP and two molecules of NADH. Phosphofructokinase is the enzyme that converts fructose 6-phosphate to fructose 1,6-biphosphate. This is irreversible, and is considered the rate-limiting step of glycolysis. In aerobic conditions, the pyruvate enters the tricarboxylic acid cycle within the mitochondria and subsequently generates ATP in a process of oxidative metabolism. (See **Figures 2.1** and **2.2**).

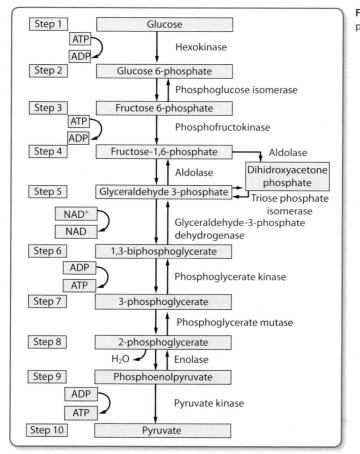

Figure 2.1 The glycolysis pathway.

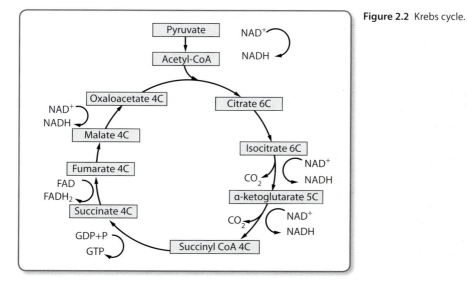

Figure 2.2 Krebs cycle.

4. B Pyruvate

Glycolysis is the metabolic pathway that converts glucose into pyruvate, which takes place in the cytoplasm of the cell. The pathway forms a sequence of 10 reactions, involving intermediary compounds at each step, which can provide entry points into the pathway. This metabolic pathway is common to both aerobic and anaerobic forms of respiration. In aerobic respiration, pyruvate then enters the tricarboxylic acid cycle, which takes place within the mitochondria. In anaerobic conditions, the pyruvate obtained from glycolysis is reduced to lactate via the action of lactate dehydrogenase. (See **Figures 2.1** and **2.2**).

5. E Tyrosine

Essential amino acids are those that cannot be synthesised directly and therefore must be obtained through dietary intake. Non-essential amino acids are those that can be synthesised without the need for dietary supplementation (**Table 2.2**).

Table 2.2 Essential and non-essential amino acids			
Essential amino acids		**Non-essential amino acids**	
Arginine	Methionine	Alanine	Glutamic acid
Histidine	Phenylalanine	Aspartic acid	Glycine
Isoleucine	Threonine	Asparagine	Proline
Leucine	Tryptophan	Cysteine	Serine
Lysine	Valine	Glutamine	Tyrosine

6. B Metabolic alkalosis

This patient has developed a metabolic alkalosis secondary to persistent vomiting and loss of hydrochloric acid from the stomach contents. Compensation occurs in the lungs by trying to retain carbon dioxide through hypoventilation. Carbon dioxide is then used for the formation of carbonic acid, reducing pH. Peripheral chemoreceptors are sensitive to pH and are stimulated by the decrease in H^+ concentration. The increase in pCO_2 leads to activation of central chemoreceptors, which are sensitive to partial pressure of carbon dioxide in the blood. This then leads to a rise in respiration rate.

7. B Acetyl coenzyme A

Acetyl coenzyme A (acetyl-CoA) is not an intermediate of the citric acid cycle [also known as the tricarboxylic acid cycle (TCA cycle) or the Krebs cycle]. Pyruvate, the final product of glycolysis, is converted to acetyl-CoA via a process of pyruvate decarboxylation by the action of pyruvate dehydrogenase. Acetyl-CoA then enters the citric acid cycle. All of the other possible answers given are different intermediates produced by the citric acid cycle (**Figure 2.2**).

8. E Separation to opposite poles

Mitosis is the process by which cells duplicate and then separate their chromosomes in order to produce identical copies of the original cell. This only occurs in eukaryotic cells. The cell spends most of its time in 'interphase', a period divided into two growth periods G1 and G2, which are separated by the 'S' phase. During the latter, the cell undergoes Swanson DNA duplication in preparation for mitosis.

Mitosis truly commences as prophase, during which there is condensation of chromatin into chromosomes. This is followed by metaphase, where sister chromatids are produced by DNA replication during the 'S' phase of interphase and then align at the cell's equatorial plane, also known as the metaphase plane. Anaphase describes the subsequent separation of the sister chromatids to opposite poles of the cell. Following this separation there is breakdown of the parent cell's nuclear membrane, which reforms around each separate set of chromosomes. Cytokinesis describes the separation of the cytoplasm, marking the final step in the formation of the daughter cells.

9. D Southern blotting

The Southern blot is a technique used to identify specific sequences of DNA amongst material containing many other DNA sequences. Developed in the 1970s by the microbiologist Edward Southern, it uses electrophoresis techniques to identify target DNA sequences. Techniques that use principles identified by Southern have been given similar nomenclature in tribute to his original methods. Northern blotting is used to identify specific RNA sequences in RNA-rich matter. Western blotting identifies specific proteins in samples using both gel electrophoresis and also immunoblotting, whereby antibodies mark the protein of interest. Eastern blotting can be considered as an extension of the Western blotting technique and detects protein post-translational modifications. Northwestern blotting is a fictional technique.

10. B Transport of cholesterol from the liver to tissues around the body

Lipoproteins form the basis of the transport of fats around the body. All lipoproteins consist of both fats and proteins in a complex consisting of a hydrophilic outer surface and a hydrophobic core. Low-density lipoproteins (LDLs) predominantly consist of cholesterol and cholesterol esters, and they transport cholesterol from the liver to tissues whose cells are expressing the LDL receptor. LDLs are often referred to as 'the bad cholesterol' due to their association with atheromatous change (blood vessels may also express LDL receptors). High-density lipoproteins (HDLs) are the smallest of the lipoproteins and are protein- and cholesterol-rich. HDLs 'collect' cholesterol from cells which are then sequestered into its hydrophobic core and carried to the liver (and steroid-producing organs such as the ovaries), where the cholesterol is released through the action of HDL receptors. Very low-density lipoproteins (VLDLs) are produced in the liver and comprise of predominantly triglycerides and cholesterol; in the blood, these VLDLs are converted to LDLs. Chylomicrons are responsible for transporting dietary fats, predominantly in the form of triglycerides from the small intestine to tissues, such as the liver and skeletal muscle for usage.

11. B Cortisol

Congenital adrenal hyperplasia (CAH) is used to describe a series of autosomal recessive conditions characterised by a deficiency in cortisol production (and in some forms aldosterone). Altered steroidogenesis results primarily in both cortisol deficiency and excess of its steroid precursors such as testosterone. In males, CAH may not be detected until after the first weeks of birth, when they may present with symptoms of a salt-wasting crisis such as severe vomiting, dehydration and appear to be shocked. This presentation is due to aldosterone and cortisol deficiency leading to biochemical imbalances such hyperkalaemia, and hyponatraemia.

In females, the most common form of CAH is typically diagnosed at the birth of a genetically female infant with ambiguous genitalia caused by fetal exposure to excessive levels of androgens. This form of CAH is caused by a deficiency in 21-hydroxylase, an enzyme involved in the conversion of progesterone and 17α-hydroxyprogesterone to the precursors of cortisol. Other forms of CAH include 11β-hydroxylase deficient CAH, which results in cortisol deficiency alongside excessive aldosterone, leading to hypertension; and 17-hydroxylase deficient CAH, which alongside excessive aldosterone is also associated with deficiency in the oestrogens leading to oligomenorrhoea and infertility.

Chapter 3

Embryology

Questions

For each question, select the single best answer from the five options listed.

1. Which one of the following constitutes the parameters for a normal sperm count?

	Volume (mL)	Motility (% progressive)	Count (million/mL)	Morphology (% normal forms)
A	2.0–5.0	20	20	< 10
B	2.0–5.0	90	20	< 20
C	2.0–5.0	40	15	< 5
D	1.0–3.0	80	60	< 10
E	1.0–3.0	90	20	< 5

2. Which of the following best describes the process of compaction?

   A   It leads to the formation of the trophoblast
   B   It leads to the formation of the cytotrophoblast
   C   It is a reaction of the chromosomes during meiosis
   D   It leads to the formation of the morula after the 16 cell stage
   E   It refers to the reaction of the sperm head on penetration of the ovum

3. Regarding germ cell layers, which of the following is correct?

   A   Endoderm: endocrine glands
   B   Endoderm: nervous system
   C   Ectoderm: most proximal layer
   D   Mesoderm: lung cells
   E   Mesoderm: skin epidermis

4. The cells of which structure form the chorionic villi?

   A   Neural crest
   B   Endoderm
   C   Primitive streak
   D   Hypoblast
   E   Extraembryonic mesoderm

5. Müllerian-inhibiting hormone inhibits the development of the paramesonephric duct.

    Where is Müllerian-inhibiting hormone secreted from?

    A   Ovarian granulosa cells
    B   Ovarian theca cells
    C   Placenta
    D   Testicular Leydig cells
    E   Testicular Sertoli cells

6. How long after fertilisation does the fetal heart start to beat?

    A   0–1 weeks
    B   2–3 weeks
    C   4–5 weeks
    D   6–7 weeks
    E   8–9 weeks

7. What structure does the embryological urachus eventually form?

    A   Inferior epigastric artery
    B   Medial umbilical ligament
    C   Median umbilical ligament
    D   Round ligament
    E   Urinary bladder

8. What embryological structure becomes the permanent/functional kidney?

    A   Guberenaculum
    B   Mesonephros
    C   Metanephros
    D   Pronephros
    E   Urachus

Answers

1. C

	Volume (mL)	Motility (% progressive)	Count (million/mL)	Morphology (% normal forms)
C	2.0–5.0	40	15	<5

On average, an ejaculate will have a volume of 2–5 mL seminal fluid. The average sperm count in this fluid is 60×10^6/mL and a low sperm count would be associated with a count of < 15 million/mL. Motility describes the action and movement of the sperm, and the proportion of which have forward motion. The progressive motility should be at least 40%. Another parameter that is used to classify sperm counts is morphology. It is normal to have some abnormal spermatozoa; the minimum acceptable percentage of semen with normal morphology is 4%.

2. D It leads to the formation of the morula after the 16 cell stage

Compaction refers to the stage of cell division when the cells flatten out and it becomes impossible to determine cell outlines. This occurs between the 16 and 32 cell stage when the embryo becomes a morula. The reaction of the sperm with the ovum is known as capacitation.

3. A Endoderm: endocrine glands

The three embryonic germ cell layers are:

- Endoderm
- Mesoderm
- Ectoderm

Each of these layers gives rise to different parts of the embryo, as summarised in **Table 3.1**.

Table 3.1 Germ cell layers		
Ectoderm	Distal layer	Nervous system
		Skin epidermis
Mesoderm	Middle layer	Muscles (cardiac, skeletal)
		Connective tissue
		Blood vessels
		Bone
		Reproductive system
Endoderm	Proximal layer	Gastrointestinal tract
		Respiratory tract
		Endocrine glands

4. E Extraembryonic mesoderm

It is the cells of the extraembryonic mesoderm that develop into the chorionic villi.

The neural crest gives rise to the nervous system and melanocytes. Endoderm is one of the germ cell layers and produces the gastrointestinal tract, respiratory tract and endocrine organs. The primitive streak develops by the end of the second week in the bilaminar embryonic disc and functions to determine symmetry of the developing embryo. The hypoblast is a part of the inner cell mass and lies beneath the epiblast. It gives rise to extraembryonic endoderm.

5. E Testicular Sertoli cells

The development of the paramesonephric ducts is controlled by the glycoprotein Müllerian-inhibiting hormone (MIH). The developing testicular Sertoli cells produce MIH from week 8, which cause the paramesonephric ducts to regress. The absence of MIH in female embryogenesis results in the development of the paramesonephric ducts, resulting in the uterus, uterine tubes and the upper two-thirds of the vagina.

6. B 2–3 weeks

The 2-week period after fertilisation is known as the pre-embryonic stage.

- Day 1 - Fertilisation occurs in the ampulla of the tubes 12–24 hours after ovulation
- Day 2 - Cleavage occurs
- Day 3 - Compaction forms the morula.
- Day 5 - Cavitation forms the blastocyst, which contains 16 cells and an inner cell and outer cell mass. It moves down the fallopian tubes to the uterine lumen.
- Day 7 - Implantation occurs when the uterine cavity is breached and decidualisation is initiated, which forms the inner cytotrophoblast and outer syncytiotrophoblast.
- Weeks 2–3 - Gastrulation results in the development of the three germ cell layers, the ectoderm, mesoderm and endoderm. The presence of the primitive streak

marks the onset of gastrulation, through which the cells migrate. The notochord is present and defines the midline from which it has an important signaling role and drives neurulation. The notochord later regress to become the nucleus pulposus of the intervertebral discs.

- Weeks 3–8 - This is the embryonic stage. Segmentation occurs, during which blocks of paraxial mesoderm become organised into somites, which are the building blocks for ribs, vertebrae or skin dermis. The fetal heart starts to beat at day 21.

7. C Median umbilical ligament

Many anatomical landmarks are remnants from important embryological structures, for example:

The gubernaculum splits into two parts; the upper and lower sections. In males, the upper part degenerates with the lower part becoming the scrotal ligament, whereas in women the upper part becomes the suspensory ligament, with the lower part becoming the round ligament.

The urachus becomes the median umbilical ligament. The medial umbilical ligament is formed from a remnant of the umbilical artery. The left umbilical vein becomes the ligamentum teres of the liver, and the right umbilical vein disappears.

The cloaca becomes the urinary bladder. The ductus arteriosus and venosus develop into the ligamentum arteriosum and venosum respectively.

8. C Metanephros

The pronephros is the first stage of embryological renal development, but by the 4th week of embryonic life, it disappears completely.

The mesonephros develops through the formation of mesonephric tubules from the embryological intermediate mesoderm. It acts as the principal excretory organ during embryological weeks 6–10. It gradually degenerates, although parts develop into the male reproductive organs.

The metanephros develops from mesonephros; it is a functional kidney from week 12, and derives from intermediate mesoderm. The ureteric bud arises as a diverticulum from the Wollfian duct close to the cloaca.

Chapter 4

Endocrinology

Questions

For each question, select the single best answer from the five options listed.

1. An 18-year-old woman presents to the gynaecology clinic for an investigation of amenorrhoea. You notice that she is overweight with hirsutism, and has both a round face and acne. After looking up recent blood tests, you notice that her plasma cortisol is high and her adrenocorticotrophic hormone (ACTH) is undetectable.

    What is the most likely cause of these results?

    A   Cushing's syndrome (adrenal origin)
    B   Cushing's syndrome (ectopic ACTH production)
    C   Cushing's syndrome (pituitary origin)
    D   Polycystic ovarian syndrome
    E   Primary adrenal failure

2. What is a site of action of antidiuretic hormone?

    A   Bowman's capsule
    B   Collecting duct
    C   Glomerulus
    D   Loop of Henle
    E   Proximal convoluted tubule

3. Prior to undergoing a routine vaginal hysterectomy for prolapse, a 72-year-old woman attends a pre-assessment clinic. Her blood pressure is found to be high and electrolytes deranged.

    Which of the following is a secondary cause of hyperaldosteronism?

    A   Conn's syndrome
    B   Diabetes insipidus
    C   Renal artery stenosis
    D   Syndrome of inappropriate antidiuretic hormone secretion
    E   Tuberculosis

4. A 60-year-old woman with a chronic disease is admitted to hospital feeling acutely unwell. She has severe diarrhoea and vomiting. She is hypotensive with a blood pressure of 85/45 mmHg. You suspect that she has Addison's disease.

Which of the following is a recognised cause of Addison's disease?

A　Diabetes insipidus
B　HIV
C　Hyperparathyroidism
D　Pregnancy
E　Sarcoidosis

5.　A 24-year-old woman is admitted to hospital for vomiting and diarrhoea at 26 weeks' gestation. Her electrolytes are deranged and fail to resolve after the acute event, and she requires admission to the high-dependency unit. You suspect Addison's disease.

Which of the following is the most appropriate initial specific test for Addison's disease?

A　Dexamethasone suppression test
B　Short adrenocorticotrophic hormone (ACTH) inhibition test
C　Short ACTH stimulation test
D　Long ACTH inhibition test
E　Long ACTH stimulation test

6.　Which is the first catecholamine to be produced in the synthesis of catecholamines?

A　Dopamine
B　Epinephrine
C　Norepinephrine
D　Phenylalanine
E　Tyrosine

7.　A 48-year-old woman is found to have persistent hypertension during a work-up for gynaecology operation. Further investigation reveals a phaeochromocytoma.

Which of the following biochemical changes is associated with phaeochromocytoma?

A　Basophilia
B　Hyperglycaemia
C　Hyperkalaemia
D　Hypocalcaemia
E　Reduced urinary catecholamines

8.　Which of the following actions is related to glucagon?

A　Decreases gluconeogenesis
B　Decreases ketone body production
C　Decreases plasma glucose
D　Increases glycogenolysis
E　Reduces lipolysis

9. A 32-year-old Asian woman is diagnosed at 28 weeks' gestation with gestational diabetes. Treatment with metformin is commenced.

   Which of the following is an insulin antagonist?

   A   Cortisol
   B   Free fatty acids
   C   Growth hormone
   D   Prolactin
   E   Somatostatin

10. A 51-year-old woman begins hormonal replacement therapy (HRT). You consider the properties of oestrogen when discussing the contraindications to HRT treatment.

    Which of the following is a property of oestrogen?

    A   Decreases bone formation
    B   Decreases circulating coagulation factors
    C   Increases bowel motility
    D   Reduce triglycerides in blood
    E   Stimulates growth of endometrium

11. A 21-year-old woman is started on the mini pill. She asks you about the possible side effects of progesterone.

    Which of the following is a property of progesterone?

    A   Increases contractility of uterine smooth muscle
    B   Increases respiratory drive
    C   Inhibits lobular alveolar development of mammary glands
    D   Promotes lactation during pregnancy
    E   Reduces bone density

12. A 32-year-old woman is referred to the gynaecology clinic with secondary amenorrhoea. Day 21 progesterone levels indicate that she is not ovulating.

    Which of the following statements best describes the events occurring at the midluteal phase of the menstrual cycle?

    A   An increase in progesterone and selective rise in follicle-stimulating hormone (FSH)
    B   High progesterone leads to low FSH and luteinising hormone (LH)
    C   Oestradiol decreases and FSH increases
    D   Oestradiol feedback becomes negative leading to LH surge
    E   Peak of LH surge

13. A 34-year-old woman undergoes regular ultrasound scans for follicle tracking having been started on clomiphene treatment.

    Which of the following statements most appropriately describes the mature ovarian follicle?

    A   Its development is primarily controlled by luteinising hormone
    B   It is surrounded by theca cells
    C   It is usually the only primary follicle to develop during each cycle
    D   It produces progesterone
    E   It reaches a diameter of 20–30 mm prior to rupture

14. A 23-year-old woman attends the gynaecology clinic after an ultrasound scan reveals multiple cysts on both ovaries. She also complains of irregular menstrual cycles and has been trying to conceive for over 1 year.

Which of the following lead to clinical manifestations of polycystic ovarian syndrome?

    A   Decrease in oestradiol levels
    B   Decrease in prolactin
    C   Decrease in testosterone and androstenedione
    D   Increase in fasting insulin
    E   Increase in sex hormone binding globulin

15. Which of the following increases sex hormone binding globulin?

    A   Growth hormone
    B   Hepatic cirrhosis
    C   Hyperprolactinaemia
    D   Hypogonadism
    E   Hypothyroidism

16. A 46-year-old woman attends the gynaecology clinic complaining of irregular, heavy periods. On taking a history, she complains of occasional hot flushes and low mood. She has had a normal pelvic ultrasound scan. You suspect that she is perimenopausal, but organise an outpatient hysteroscopy and some blood tests.

Which of the following statements is most accurate in regard to the menopause?

    A   The average age of the menopause in the UK is 53 years
    B   Oestradiol levels can be used to aid diagnosis of the climacteric/menopause
    C   Follicle-stimulating hormone and luteinising hormone fall
    D   Progesterone levels rise
    E   Urogenital atrophy is caused by falling levels of oestrogens

17. An 8-year-old girl attends the emergency department with vaginal bleeding. Sexual abuse is ruled out. On examination it is noted that she has significant breast tissue and is taller than average for her age. Differential diagnosis includes precocious puberty.

Which of the following statements regarding pubertal changes in the female is most accurate?

    A   Thelarche follows menarche
    B   Adrenarche precedes thelarche

    C Ovulation is established from the first period
    D Menarche before the age of 12 years is considered precocious puberty
    E Changes occur in response to increasingly regular pulses of gonadotrophin-releasing hormone

18. A 28-year-old woman is seen in the antenatal clinic at 34 weeks' gestation. She has gestational diabetes and her blood sugar control is suboptimal despite metformin treatment. The abdominal circumference of the fetus is over the 97th centile at her most recent growth scan. The consultant decides to start insulin injections.

    Which statement most accurately describes the function of insulin?

    A Increases lipolysis
    B Decreases gluconeogenesis
    C Decreases glycogen synthetase
    D Increases ketogenesis
    E Activates glycogen phosphorylase

19. A 10-year-old girl with short stature presents at the outpatient clinic. Differential diagnoses may be related to conditions leading to a lack of growth hormone.

    Which of the following most accurately describes the function of growth hormone?

    A It is primarily catabolic in action
    B Is released in a pulsatile manner every 90 minutes
    C Inhibits protein synthesis
    D Stimulates lipolysis
    E Is released in lower quantities in patients with anorexia nervosa

20. A 25-year-old primiparous woman is admitted in spontaneous labour to the birth centre, but she has slow progress in the first stage. She is transferred to the labour ward for assessment and you make the decision to start her on a syntocinon infusion as her contractions are only occurring twice every 10 minutes.

    With regards to oxytocin, which of the following is true?

    A It is stored in the hypothalamus
    B It acts via a G-protein-coupled receptor
    C It is a decapeptide
    D It is responsible for milk production
    E It has an identical structure to vasopressin

21. With regards to ovarian steroidogenesis, which of the following is true?

    A Progesterone is produced by the ovarian theca cells only
    B Testosterone is produced by the ovarian theca cells only
    C Oestradiol is produced by the ovarian theca cells
    D Theca cells have follicle-stimulating hormone (FSH) receptors
    E Granulosa cells are responsive to FSH only

22. A woman undergoes in vitro fertilisation (IVF) for age-related female factor primary infertility.

    Regarding the female reproductive system, which of the following statements most accurately describes the oocyte?

    A   Primary oocytes are arrested at first mitotic division until ovulation
    B   Completion of first meiotic division occurs in response to the luteinising hormone surge
    C   First polar body is found in the sperm head
    D   Completion of the first meiotic division leads to the primary oocyte
    E   Second meiotic division is not completed until after implantation

23. Regarding adrenal function during pregnancy, which of the following is most accurate?

    A   Cortisol levels decrease throughout pregnancy
    B   Cortisol-binding globulin synthesis increases
    C   Aldosterone levels fall
    D   Angiotensin II levels fall
    E   Renin levels are unchanged

Answers

---

1. A Cushing's syndrome (adrenal origin)

Cushing's syndrome as a result of an adrenal tumour leads to increased plasma cortisol and very low levels of ACTH, as shown in **Table 4.1**.

Table 4.1 Levels of cortisol and adrenocorticotrophic hormone (ACTH) in various pathologies

	Cortisol	ACTH
Normal	Low – midnight High – 0800	Not raised
Primary adrenal failure	Low	High
Steroid therapy	Variable	Variable (may be normal or very low)
Cushing's (adrenal origin)	High	Low (undetectable)
Cushing's (pituitary origin)	High	High
Cushing's (ectopic ACTH production)	High	Very high

---

2. B Collecting duct

Antidiuretic hormone (ADH) or vasopressin is a peptide hormone that helps to regulate water homeostasis. It is released from the posterior pituitary in response to increased osmolality of plasma and acts on the distal tubule of the kidney to increase water absorption via insertion of aquaporins water channels into the membrane. By increasing the water reabsorption of the kidney, the osmolality of the urine is increased. Nephrogenic diabetes insipidus is caused when the kidney become unresponsive to ADH. Acquired forms of nephrogenic diabetes insipidus may be triggered by hypokalaemia, pregnancy, hydronephrosis or drugs (e.g. lithium).

---

3. C Renal artery stenosis

Primary hyperaldosteronism is the excess production of aldosterone, independent of the renin–angiotensin–aldosterone system. Features suggestive of hyperaldosteronism include hypertension with hypokalaemia and alkalosis. More than 50% of cases are due to Conn's syndrome, a unilateral adrenocortical adenoma. The most appropriate form of treatment in this case is laparoscopic removal of the tumour. Other causes of primary hyperaldosteronism include bilateral adrenal hyperplasia; spironolactone therapy is often successful in treating these cases. Secondary causes of hyperaldosteronism include renal artery stenosis which leads to a perceived hypoperfusion of the kidney and increased secretion of renin and aldosterone. The hypertension is often refractory to treatment, especially with angiotensin converting enzyme inhibitors. The syndrome of inappropriate antidiuretic hormone (ADH) secretion has multiple causes including small cell carcinoma of the lung, stroke, encephalitis and postoperatively. Excessive secretion of ADH leads to hyponatraemia and fluid overload.

4. B HIV

Addison's disease is caused by primary adrenocortical insufficiency, most commonly with an autoimmune cause. It has an incidence of approximately 1/100,000 and is therefore relatively rare. Autoimmunity may lead to antibodies against the adrenal gland and may be associated with other autoimmune diseases, including thyroid disease, pernicious anaemia and diabetes. Other causes include tuberculosis and acute bleeding into the adrenal gland (Waterhouse–Friderichsen syndrome).

HIV is now a common cause of Addison's disease in areas, where HIV is prevalent.

Sarcoidosis is not classically known to cause Addison's disease.

5. C Short ACTH stimulation test

Addison's disease does not become apparent until 90% of the gland is destroyed.

Hyperkalaemia and hyponatraemia are usual initial laboratory findings with symptoms of fatigue, abdominal pain, weakness, constipation, hyperpigmentation and weight loss. In severe cases of Addisonian crisis there may be postural hypotension, confusion. Diagnosis is usually confirmed with the short adrenocorticotrophic hormone (ACTH) stimulation test (also known as the Synacthen test), when plasma cortisol levels are tested before and after synthetic ACTH. The long ACTH stimulation test may be used once the results of the initial short test are noted to be abnormal. In treating Addison's disease, it is essential to replace glucocorticoids (hydrocortisone) and mineralocorticoids (fludrocortisone). Hyperpigmentation is caused by an excess of ACTH which is released by the pituitary in order to trigger production of cortisol by the adrenal gland. In secondary adrenal failure, there is low ACTH due to deficient corticotrophin-releasing hormone release by the hypothalamus.

6. A Dopamine

Catecholamines are derived from the amino acid tyrosine and have a half-life in the circulation of a few minutes. The first step is the conversion of tyrosine to L-dopa by the enzyme tyrosine hydroxylase, which is the rate-limiting step in the synthetic pathway. Dopamine is the first catecholamine to be produced, followed by norepinephrine and epinephrine. Catecholamines are degraded by catechol-O-methyltransferase (COMT) or monoamine oxidases (MAO).

7. B Hyperglycaemia

Phaeochromocytoma is a tumour that produces catecholamines and is a rare cause of resistant hypertension. It is usually found in the adrenal medulla, but 10%

are found elsewhere. Other symptoms include palpitations and psychological symptoms. Investigation may reveal glycosuria in up to one-third of patients.

Hyperglycaemia is caused primarily by the stimulation of lipolysis because of catecholamine production. Stimulation at β-adrenergic receptors leads to glycogenolysis and gluconeogenesis. During attacks, thirty per cent of patients have glycosuria. Investigations to establish a diagnosis of phaeochromocytoma include 24-hour urine collection for vanillylmandelic acid, which is a catecholamine metabolite. Hyperkalaemia and basophilia are not typically associated with phaeochromocytoma.

8. D Increases glycogenolysis

Glucagon is a polypeptide composed of 21 amino acids. It is synthesised by the islet cells of the pancreas and is essential for the control of glucose homeostasis. Secretion is stimulated by low glucose states and is inhibited if blood sugars are raised. In states of low blood glucose, there is an increase in the activity of the sympathetic nervous system which causes an increase in circulating adrenaline. This in turn stimulates the β-adrenoreceptors and leads to an increase in glucagon. The main action of glucagon is to increase blood glucose and leads to a breakdown in stored fat and protein; it acts mainly on the liver.

9. E Somatostatin

Insulin is a peptide hormone synthesised and secreted by the β cells of the islet of Langerhans of the pancreas. It is secreted as a prohormone, which is converted to an active hormone by proteolytic cleavage of the C-peptide. Insulin is the main hormone controlling the blood glucose levels. Insulin is released in response to increased amino acids, free fatty acids and gastric hormone which are released in response to eating, including cholecystokinin, gastrin and secretin. Insulin release is inhibited by adrenaline and somatostatin.

10. E Stimulates growth of endometrium

Oestrogen causes the following effects on:

Coagulation

- Increases circulating coagulating factors, including plasminogen, factors II, VII, IX, X. Increase antithrombin III

Lipids

- Increases high-density lipoproteins
- Increases triglycerides
- Reduces low-density lipoproteins

Gastrointestinal

- Reduces bowel motility

Structural

- Stimulates endometrial growth
- Increases discharge and lubrication
- Increases bone formation
- Promotes formation of secondary sexual characteristics

Fluid balance

- Increases salt and water retention

11. B Increases respiratory drive

Progesterone is a C-21 steroid hormone derived from cholesterol. As well as increasing respiratory drive, it reduces bowel motility and increases basal body temperature. Levels increase during the luteal phase of the menstrual cycle in preparation for fertilisation of the ovum. If pregnancy does not occur, the corpus luteum degenerates and levels of progesterone fall. Progesterone protects the endometrium from cancer.

12. C Oestradiol decreases and FSH increases

During each menstrual cycle, up to ten secondary follicles are recruited. One will become a dominant follicle and the rest will regress. There is pulsatile production of gonadotrophin-releasing hormones from the hypothalamus and subsequent release of follicle-stimulating hormone (FSH) and luteinising hormone (LH) from the pituitary. The developing follicle produces oestrogen under the influence of FSH. LH acts on the thecal cells of the ovary to produce androgens. There is feedback from the ovarian hormones to the pituitary and hypothalamus. The follicle stimulates the ovary to produce oestrogen which stimulates production of the glandular endometrium. Oestrogen levels increase, and 14 days before the onset of menstruation they become high enough to trigger a surge of LH which in turn stimulates ovulation. Once the egg has been released, the corpus luteum causes increased production of progesterone and subsequent proliferation of endometrium. If fertilisation does not occur, hormones levels fall as a result of the failing corpus luteum and menstruation begins.

13. B It is surrounded by theca cells

A layer of thecal cells surrounds the mature follicle once it has reached the secondary stage with two layers of granulosa cells. Both layers of cells serve to protect the developing follicle. During development, an oocyte will grow up to 120 μm in diameter. Development is controlled primarily by follicle-stimulating hormone rather than luteinising hormone, and it does not produce progesterone.

14. D Increase in fasting insulin

Polycystic ovary syndrome (PCOS) is the most common endocrine disturbance affecting women. It can be familial. Signs and symptoms vary amongst women and even in an individual over time. Clinical symptoms range from obesity, to menstrual irregularities, to subfertility, hirsutism, and acne. Elevations in insulin are common in both underweight and obese women with PCOS. It is thought that the insulin stimulates androgen secretion. There appears to be an insulin resistance in these women who then have an increased risk of developing diabetes

15. C Hyperprolactinaemia

Sex hormone-binding globulin (SHBG) is synthesised in the liver. 80% of testosterone is bound to SHBG, 19% to albumin and 1% is unbound. Biological effects of circulating androgens depend primarily on the unbound fraction. Its production is decreased by androgens and insulin. On the other hand, oestrogen increases the production of SHBG and hence hirsutism is improved by taking the oral contraceptive pill during pregnancy.

16. E Urogenital atrophy is caused by falling levels of oestrogens

The menopause is a retrospective diagnosis made when a woman has been amenorrhoeic for at least one year. The 'climacteric' encompasses the time from when a woman may experience classic menopausal symptoms, such as hot flushes, together with menstrual irregularity, up to the cessation of periods. With age there is an ovarian atresia, with fewer ovulatory cycles; this leads to lower levels of oestrogen production. Follicle-stimulating hormone (FSH) and luteinising hormone (LH) levels are subsequently raised in an attempt to increase oestrogen levels. Associated with the reduction in overall levels of oestradiol is the failure of endometrial proliferation and subsequent cessation of menstruation. Measuring FSH levels can be a useful investigation with levels above 30 IU/L aiding diagnosis of the menopause. The measurement of oestrodiol levels is not a useful tool in the diagnosis of the menopause as levels may fluctuate because of the continued peripheral conversion of androstenedione to oestrogens by ovarian tissue, adipose tissues, the liver and the adrenal glands. Oestrone is the predominant form of oestrogen postmenopausally. There is no role for the measurement of LH, oestrogen, testosterone or progesterone levels (**Table 4.2**).

Table 4.2 Hormones and the menopause	
Hormone	**Menopausal levels**
Follicle-stimulating hormone	Increased
Luteinising hormone	Increased
Oestrogens	Overall levels of oestradiol decrease
	Oestrogens still made peripheral conversion in tissues
	Oestrone predominant postmenopausal oestrogen
Testosterone	Unchanged
Progesterone	Decreased

17. E Changes occur in response to increasingly regular pulses of gonadotrophin-releasing hormone

On average puberty in the UK occurs at around 12 years old; it entails a series of changes in endocrine function and physical appearance which accompany the change to adulthood. In females, thelarche is the process of breast development that follows a growth spurt. It usually precedes adrenarche, the process of pubic hair development, which is followed by menarche, the commencement of menstruation. Menarche prior to the age of 10 years is considered precocious.

Failure to commence by the age of 16 years warrants further investigation. Tanner staging is a means of grading pubertal breast and pubic hair development in female; it is also used in males to grade pubic hair and testicular development.

Tanner staging is graded I to IV, the latter representing the adult form. Puberty is associated with the commencement of gonadotrophin-releasing hormone pulses in late childhood, which become increasingly regular, gradually changing from nocturnal pulses to pulses occurring every 90 minutes. These pulses stimulate the production of follicle-stimulating and luteinising hormones with subsequent production of oestrogen and testosterone. Growth hormone levels are increased during puberty and its actions, mediated by insulin-like growth factor-1 are thought to be responsible for the pubertal growth spurt.

18. B Decreases gluconeogenesis

The overall function of insulin is to decrease hepatic output of glucose. This occurs via the following mechanisms:

- Promotion of glycogen synthesis
- This increases glycogen synthetase (muscle and liver) and inhibits glycogen phosphorylase
- Decrease gluconeogenesis
- Suppress lipolysis
- This inhibits triglyceride lipase and increases fatty acid synthetase
- Suppress ketogenesis
- This inhibit carnitine palmitoyltransferase and increases acetyl coenzyme A carboxylase

19. D Stimulates lipolysis

Growth hormone (GH) is a peptide and consists of 191 amino acids. The locus for the growth hormone gene is on chromosome 17. It has a molecular weight of around 21,000 daltons and is structurally similar to both prolactin and human placental lactogen. It is secreted from the anterior pituitary gland somatotrophs in response to GH-releasing hormone. Somatostatin is a direct inhibitor of GH. GH release stimulates lipolysis, gluconeogenesis and the synthesis of insulin-like growth factors. Insulin growth factors stimulate bone growth and protein synthesis in muscles.

GH release is stimulated by GH-releasing hormone and inhibited by somatostatin, both of which are produced by the hypothalamus. The action of GH is principally one of the anabolism, which is reflected in its role in lipolysis and its anti-insulinic properties. GH is secreted in higher levels during puberty when more frequent pulsatile release occurs. The growth-promoting actions of GH are mediated by insulin-like growth factor-1.

20. B It acts via a G-protein-coupled receptor

Oxytocin is produced by the supraoptic and paraventricular nuclei of the anterior hypothalamus and then transported to the posterior pituitary gland where it is stored for release. It is a nonapeptide, which consists of nine amino acids. It has a very similar structure to vasopressin (antidiuretic hormone), another nonapeptide also stored in the posterior pituitary gland. Oxytocin is involved in the release of breast milk, rather than its production. It is involved in the 'let down' reflex whereby stimulation of the nipples by the suckling infant leads to release of oxytocin, which then leads to milk ejection. Prolactin is responsible for milk production. Oxytocin also plays an important role in the contraction of uterine muscle during labour.

21. B Testosterone is produced by the ovarian theca cells only

The production of steroid hormones by the ovary depends on the menstrual cycle. Progesterone is produced by the ovarian theca and granulosa cells and is produced mainly during the luteal phase of the menstrual cycle. During the follicular phase of the cycle, it is mainly oestrogen that is produced. Testosterone is produced by the theca only. Oestradiol, the end product of steroidogenesis, is produced only by the granulosa cells. In the ovarian follicles, theca cells have receptors for luteinising hormone (LH) and not follicle-stimulating hormone (FSH). Granulosa cells have receptors for FSH and for LH later on.

22. B Completion of first meiotic division occurs in response to the luteinising hormone surge

Oogonia fill the ovaries during fetal life, and these primordial germ cells divide by mitosis until shortly before birth. No further oocytes are produced after birth and at this time each female has approximately one million oocytes. Primary oocytes are contained in the ovary of the fetus and arrested after the first meiotic division until ovulation. Although the oogonia are arrested in the first prophase stage of meiosis, they are surrounded by a layer of granulosa cells. Oocytes surrounded by this protective layer are known as primordial follicles and are located in the cortex of the ovary. When the luteinising hormone surge occurs, the dominant follicle completes this first meiotic division to become a secondary oocyte. The first polar body is found in the ovum and contains half the chromosomes. The second meiotic division is not completed until fertilisation.

23. B Cortisol-binding globulin synthesis increases

All levels of adrenal function are increased in pregnancy, and this includes corticotrophin-releasing factor. Synthesis of both cortisol and cortisol-binding globulin is increased. Levels of aldosterone, angiotensin II and renin increase. The trophoblast increases the amount of ACTH produced with overall maternal levels remaining stable.

Chapter 5

Statistics and epidemiology

Questions

For each question, select the single best answer from the five options listed.

1. Which of the following is a quality of the median of a data set?
    A   It is distorted by skewed data
    B   It is always higher than the mean
    C   It is obtained by dividing the sum of the data set by the number of values in the data set
    D   It is the middle value in a ranked set of data
    E   It is the most frequently occurring value in a data set

2. What is the World Health Organization's definition of the perinatal mortality rate?
    A   The number of deaths in the first week of life per 1,000 live births
    B   The number of stillbirths and deaths in the first week of life per 1,000 live births
    C   The number of stillbirths and deaths in the first week of life per 10,000 live births
    D   The number of stillbirths and deaths in the first week of life per 100,000 live births
    E   The number of stillbirths and deaths in the first 28 days of life per 1,000 deliveries

3. The 'Mothers and Babies: Reducing Risk through Audits and Confidential Enquiries across the UK' (MBRRACE-UK) programme defines maternal mortality as:
    A   The number of deaths per 1000 pregnancies
    B   The number of deaths per 100,000 pregnancies
    C   The number of direct and indirect deaths per 100,000 mortalities
    D   The number of direct and indirect deaths per 10,000 mortalities
    E   The number of direct and indirect deaths per 100,000 pregnancies

4. Within what time frame does the 'Mothers and Babies: Reducing Risk through Audits and Confidential Enquiries across the UK' (MBRRACE-UK) programme consider maternal death to have occurred?

A   During pregnancy
B   During pregnancy or within 28 days of the end of the pregnancy
C   During pregnancy or within 42 days of the end of the pregnancy
D   Within 14 days of the end of the pregnancy
E   Within 42 days of the end of the pregnancy

5.   An antenatal clinic undertakes a month-long study looking at the diastolic blood pressure of women at their antenatal booking visit. The data collected has a normal Gaussian distribution.

The following values are obtained:

N = 93

Mean diastolic blood pressure = 82 mmHg

Variance = 9

What is the standard deviation of the data set?

A   2
B   3
C   5
D   12
E   18

6.   One hundred women with postmenopausal bleeding have pelvic ultrasound scans to measure endometrial thickness and have a Pipelle biopsy taken.

The findings of the scan – normal or thickened endometrial thickness – and the subsequent histology of the Pipelle biopsies – normal or showing endometrial cancer – are shown in the table below.

Pelvic scan result	Endometrial cancer on Pipelle (n)	Normal endometrium on Pipelle (n)	Total (n)
Abnormal	10	8	18
Normal	2	80	82
Total	12	88	100

What is the sensitivity (to the closest per cent) of the pelvic scan in detecting endometrial cancer?

A   25%
B   55%
C   83%
D   91%
E   98%

7.   One hundred women with postmenopausal bleeding have pelvic ultrasound scans to measure endometrial thickness and have a Pipelle biopsy taken.

The findings of the scan, normal or thickened endometrial thickness, and the subsequent histology of the Pipelle biopsies, normal or showing endometrial cancer, are shown in the table below.

Pelvic scan result	Endometrial cancer on Pipelle (n)	Normal endometrium on Pipelle (n)	Total (n)
Abnormal	10	8	18
Normal	2	80	82
Total	12	88	100

What is the specificity (to the closest per cent) of the pelvic scan in detecting endometrial cancer?

A   25%
B   55%
C   83%
D   91%
E   98%

8. With regards to screening tests in relation to the table below, how would you correctly calculate the positive likelihood ratio?

	Diagnostic test positive	Diagnostic test negative
Screening test positive	a	c
Screening test negative	b	d

A   [a / (a + c)] / {1– [b / (b + d)]}
B   [b / (b + d)] / {1– [a / (a + c)]}
C   [d / (c + d)] / {1– [a / (a + b)]}
D   [a / (a + b)] / {1– [d / (c + d)]}
E   (a / b) / (a / c)

9. One hundred women with polycystic ovarian syndrome had their BMI measured. A summary of the results is given below:

Range = 18.0 – 38.0

Mean average value = 28.1

Median average value = 28.5

Mode average value = 29

Standard deviation = 10

What is the 95% confidence interval for this group?

A   18.0–38.0
B   18.1–38.1

   C   24.1–32.1
   D   26.1–30.1
   E   27.1–30.1

10. Your department wishes to investigate the average birthweight of term infants born to gestational diabetic women. At the end of the data collection period, there are two groups with two corresponding mean birthweight values. Given that no assumption for normal distribution can be made for these groups, what non-parametric statistical test should be used to compare the means of the two groups?

   A   Pearson's correlation co-efficient
   B   Wilcoxon signed rank test
   C   Mann-Whitney test
   D   Independent student t-test
   E   Friedman test

Answers

1. D It is the middle value in a ranked set of data

The median is one of the terms used to describe an 'average' of a set of data. The median should not be confused with the mode, which refers to the most frequently occurring value in a data set. It also differs from the mean, which is calculated by dividing the sum of the data set by the number of values in the data set. An advantage of using the median is that it is not influenced by outliers or skewed data, both of which can affect the mean of a data set. The median figure in a data set may be higher or lower than the mean.

2. B The number of stillbirths and deaths in the first week of life per 1,000 live births

The World Health Organization currently defines the perinatal mortality rate as the number of stillbirths and deaths in the first week of life per 1,000 live births (in a given period). It should not be confused with neonatal mortality, which is the number of deaths in the first completed 28 days of life per 1,000 live births. Perinatal mortality can be an important contributor to the overall neonatal mortality rate of a population.

World Health Organization. Health Status Statistics. Switzerland: WHO Press 2014.

3. E The number of direct and indirect deaths per 100,000 pregnancies

The 'Mothers and Babies: Reducing Risk through Audits and Confidential Enquiries across the UK' programme considers maternal mortality to be the number of direct and indirect deaths per 100,000 pregnancies. Direct causes of maternal mortality are those that result from obstetric complications and include sepsis, haemorrhage, pre-eclampsia/eclampsia and amniotic fluid embolism. Indirect causes are those that are not caused by obstetric complications but were made worse due to the physiological changes associated with pregnancy. These indirect causes may include conditions that were pre-existing or were diagnosed during pregnancy. Indirect causes of maternal mortality include conditions such as cardiac disease, diabetes, epilepsy and suicide.

Knight M, Kenyon S, Brocklehurst P, Neilson J, Shakespeare J, Kurinczuk JJ (Eds.) on behalf of MBRRACE-UK. Saving Lives, Improving Mothers' Care – Lessons learned to inform future maternity care from the UK and Ireland Confidential Enquiries into Maternal Deaths and Morbidity 2009–12. Oxford: University of Oxford, 2014.

4. C During pregnancy or within 42 days of the end of the pregnancy

According to the 'Mothers and Babies: Reducing Risk through Audits and Confidential Enquiries across the UK' programme, a maternal death is one that has occurred during pregnancy or within 42 days of the end of the pregnancy. The cause of the death should be related to either pregnancy or a pre-existing condition made worse due to the physiological changes associated with pregnancy. Accidental deaths are not included. Deaths may be due to direct or indirect causes. Direct causes are those that are of a direct obstetric nature, i.e. eclampsia, as opposed to indirect causes that do not have a direct obstetric cause but relate to conditions that have become more severe in pregnancy.

Knight M, Kenyon S, Brocklehurst P, Neilson J, Shakespeare J, Kurinczuk JJ (Eds.) on behalf of MBRRACEUK. Saving Lives, Improving Mothers' Care - Lessons learned to inform future maternity care from the UK and Ireland Confidential Enquiries into Maternal Deaths and Morbidity 2009–12. Oxford: University of Oxford, 2014.

5. B 3

The standard deviation of the data set is a measure of how evenly the data is spread around the mean. All the information required to calculate the standard deviation for the data set is given. The simple calculation of taking the square root of the variance is all that is required to obtain the standard deviation. Any other values given are distracters and can be ignored.

Worked answer:

Variance = 9

Square root of 9 = 3

Therefore, the standard deviation = 3

6. C 83%

The sensitivity of a test, in this case the pelvic ultrasound, refers to the proportion of individuals with the disease in question that were correctly identified by the test. In this study, this can be considered as the proportion of women who were found on Pipelle biopsy to have endometrial cancer, who were correctly identified as having an abnormal pelvic ultrasound. The specificity should be as close to 100% as possible. Sensitivity is calculated by taking the number of subjects diagnosed by the screening test and dividing it by the overall number of individuals with the condition (whether detected by the screening test or not). To give a percentage, the result is multiplied by 100.

Worked answer:

Sensitivity = endometrial cancer (with abnormal ultrasound) / endometrial cancer (with abnormal ultrasound) + endometrial cancer (with normal ultrasound) x 100

10 / (10 + 2) = 0.83

0.83 x 100 = 83%

7. D 91%

The specificity of a test refers to the proportion of individuals who were confirmed not to have the disease who were correctly identified as normal by the test. In this scenario, it refers to the proportion of individuals without endometrial cancer who had a normal pelvic ultrasound scan. In similarity to sensitivity, ideally the specificity of a test should be as close to 100% as possible. Specificity can be calculated by dividing the number of individuals without the condition who had a normal result from the initial screening test by the total number of individuals without the condition (including those who initially had an abnormal initial test).

Worked answer:

Specificity = not diagnosed with endometrial cancer (with normal ultrasound) / not diagnosed with endometrial cancer (with normal ultrasound) + not diagnosed with endometrial cancer (with abnormal ultrasound) x 100

80 / (80 + 8) = 80 / 88 = 0.91

0.91 x 100 = 91%

8. D [a / (a + b)] / {1 − [d / (c + d)]}

Test results can be positive or negative, so there are at least two likelihood ratios for each test. The positive likelihood ratio tells us how much to increase the probability of the disease if the test is positive. The general formula for calculating likelihood ratios is probability that an individual with the disease has the test result divided by probability that an individual without the disease has the test result. You can also calculate the positive and negative likelihood ratio using sensitivity and specificity.

Positive likelihood result = sensitivity / (1 − specificity)

Negative likelihood result= (1 − sensitivity) / specificity

9. D 26.1 − 30.1

The confidence interval (CI) is calculated using the mean and the standard error of the mean (SEM). The level of confidence required determines the number of SEMs either side of the mean the confidence interval will be. The multiples of SEM for corresponding confidence levels is shown below.

Confidence Level	Multiples of SE
90%	1.65
95%	1.96, usually rounded to 2
98%	2.33
99%	2.58

E.g. 95% CI = mean +/− 2×SEM

The SEM quantifies how close your estimate is to the true mean of the population. It is a method of comparing the sample mean with the population mean. SEM is the standard deviation (SD) divided by the square root of sample size (n).

Thus, the SEM is always smaller than the SD.

So in this example question:

SEM = SD / Square root of 100

So SEM = 10 / 10 = 1

So 95% CI = 28.1 +/− 2×1 = 26.1 − 30.1

10. C Mann–Whitney Test

Tests for measuring normality of distribution		
Accurate test of distribution	Kolmogorov–Smirnov	
Method of estimating distribution	Histogram	
Tests for comparing different variables and groups		
	Tests for parametric data	**Tests for non-parametric data**
To compare the results between two separate groups	Independent student t–test	Mann–Whitney U
To compare results between two paired samples	Paired student t-test	Wilcoxon signed rank
To compare three or more measurements on one subject	Repeated ANOVA	Friedman
To compare one variable between three or more separate variables	One-way ANOVA	Kruskal Wallis
Relationship between variables		
Relationship between 2 continuous variables	Pearson coefficient	Spearman coefficient
	+/− 1.0 = exact positive/negative correlation	
For small numbers categorical/ordinal data	Yates	

Chapter 6

Genetics

Questions

For each question, select the single best answer from the five options listed.

1. A woman presents to the labour ward at approximately 40 weeks' gestation in spontaneous labour. She is unbooked and has received no antenatal care. On abdominal palpation, she feels large of her reported gestational age. A small male baby is born by emergency caesarean section due to fetal distress. He is found to have microcephaly, a prominent occiput, a cleft lip and palate, clenched hands and polydactyl. Soon after birth, he has apnoeic episodes and has difficulty feeding.

   What chromosomal abnormality is the most likely cause of this baby's presentation?

   A   Microdeletion of chromosome 15
   B   Microdeletion of chromosome 22
   C   Trisomy 13
   D   Trisomy 18
   E   Trisomy 21

2. A 32-year-old woman is 15 weeks pregnant in her second pregnancy. She opts to have antenatal screening and has blood taken as part of the quadruple test. The result shows reduced levels of α-fetoprotein and unconjugated oestriol with elevated β-human chorionic gonadotrophin.

   Which of the following is the most likely explanation for the screening results?

   A   Down's syndrome
   B   Edwards' syndrome
   C   Multiple pregnancy
   D   Neural tube defect
   E   Normal pregnancy

3. A 39-year-old multiparous woman is 13 weeks pregnant. She has serum screening as part of the combined test. Analysis shows an elevated level of α-fetoprotein and a normal level of pregnancy-associated plasma protein A.

   What diagnosis are the screening results suggestive of?

   A   Down's syndrome
   B   Edwards' syndrome

C   Multiple pregnancy
D   Neural tube defect
E   Normal pregnancy

4. A 37-year-old primiparous woman is 14 weeks pregnant. Following serum
    screening, the pregnancy is found to have an increased risk of trisomy 21. She
    wishes to have further testing to confirm whether the fetus is affected.

    In view of her current gestation, what is the most appropriate diagnostic test?

    A   Amniocentesis
    B   Cell-free fetal DNA sampling
    C   Chorionic villus sampling
    D   Cordocentesis
    E   Nuchal translucency imaging

5. A 29-year-old woman seeks genetic counselling as she has a number of her female
    relatives who have had either breast or ovarian cancer. Both her mother and her
    sister have been diagnosed with breast cancer. DNA sequencing subsequently
    shows that she carries a mutated form of the BRCA1 gene.

    Via which mode of inheritance is the BRCA1 gene mutation transmitted?

    A   Autosomal dominant inheritance
    B   Autosomal recessive inheritance
    C   Mitochondrial inheritance
    D   X-linked dominant inheritance
    E   X-linked recessive inheritance

6. A 34-year-old woman delivers a male baby with Down's syndrome. Chromosomal
    analysis following his birth is suggestive of familial Down's syndrome.

    What chromosomal event best describes the aetiology of familial Down's
    syndrome?

    A   Microdeletion
    B   Nonsense mutation
    C   Reciprocal translocation
    D   Robertsonian translocation
    E   Triplet repeat expansion

7. Both individuals in a couple are both known to carry the trait for a
    haemoglobinopathy. They decline any invasive testing when they conceive their
    first pregnancy. At an anomaly scan at 20 weeks' gestation the fetus is found to
    have severe hydrops fetalis. In utero death occurs at 22 weeks' gestation.

    What is the most likely cause of the fetal demise?

    A   Alpha-thalassaemia with deletion of 4 α-globin genes
    B   Beta-thalassaemia major
    C   Glucose-6-dehydrogenase deficiency
    D   Haemoglobin H disease
    E   Sickle cell disease

Answers

1. D Trisomy 18

This baby has Edwards' syndrome, also known as trisomy 18. The syndrome is caused by an extra copy of chromosome 18, which is created due an error in meiotic dysjunction. In addition to true trisomy 18, individuals may be mosaic for trisomy 18, which is where some of their cells possess an extra copy of chromosome 18 because of a translocation defect. Trisomy 18 can be detected as part of antenatal screening, for instance by the quadruple test, but in the absence of antenatal care it may not be detected until delivery. Both polyhydramnios and oligohydramnios may be observed in these pregnancies, the former as a possible indicator of defective fetal swallowing, and the latter reflecting abnormalities in the renal tract. There may also be intrauterine growth restriction.

The appearance of the baby typifies many of the features of a baby with trisomy 18. Other associated features include rocker-bottom feet, micro penis, radial aplasia and low-set ears. There is gross delay in psychomotor development and the rare individuals who survive infancy typically have severe intellectual disability.

2. A Down's syndrome

Trisomy 21, also known as Down's syndrome, is one of a number of conditions that may be screened for by using serum markers as part of the quadruple test. Reduced serum α-fetoprotein (AFP) is associated with pregnancies affected by Down's syndrome. AFP is produced by the fetal liver and yolk sac. Reduced levels of AFP are thought to be secondary to the smaller size of fetuses affected by Down's syndrome. Beta-human chorionic gonadotrophin levels are often elevated in Down's syndrome pregnancies. The quadruple test does not aim to provide a definitive diagnosis, but is a screening test with both false positive and false negative results.

3. D Neural tube defect

The combined test uses serum markers, together with fetal nuchal translucency measurement, in order to obtain an estimate as to how likely it is that a particular fetus is affected by a chromosomal or genetic disorder. Alpha-fetoprotein (AFP) is produced by the fetal liver and yolk sac. High levels of AFP are suggestive of neural tube defects, such as spina bifida, or more rarely anencephaly. This raised level is a consequence of the flow of AFP from the open neural tube of the fetus into the amniotic fluid (and secondarily maternal serum). Pregnancy-associated plasma protein A (PAPP-A) is produced by the fetus and also by the placenta. Reduced levels of PAPP-A in maternal serum can be suggestive of a fetus with an aneuploidy, such as Down's syndrome. Intrauterine growth restriction has also been associated with reduced levels of PAPP-A.

4. C Chorionic villus sampling

Chorionic villus sampling can be performed from 11 weeks' gestation and provides a means of culturing fetal placental tissue in order to determine fetal karyotyping.

Amniocentesis involves the aspiration of fetal cells found in amniotic fluid in order to perform chromosomal analysis and should ideally be performed from 15 weeks' gestation. Cordocentesis involves the sampling of fetal blood from the umbilical vein in order to perform chromosomal analysis; it may also be used to detect fetal infection and anaemia. Although currently not widely used, cell-free fetal DNA sampling detects naturally occurring fetal DNA and RNA in maternal blood. This technique can be used in the determination of fetal sex and rhesus status, and to screen for paternally-inherited dominant single gene disorders. In the future, this technique may be used to detect other genetic diseases as well as fetal aneuploidies. Nuchal translucency imaging using ultrasound is a screening test for fetal abnormalities as a thickened nuchal fold is associated with aneuploidies such as Turner's and Down's syndromes.

5. A Autosomal dominant inheritance

Several breast cancer susceptibility genes have been identified, including the *BRCA1* and *BRCA2* genes. The *BRCA1* gene is found on chromosome 17, whereas the *BRCA2* gene is found on chromosome 13. Both the *BRCA1* and *BRCA2* genes are in fact tumour suppressor genes which code for the DNA repair proteins BRCA1 protein and BRCA2 protein. Mutations in each gene lead to a defective form of the protein, with the consequence of increased tumorigenesis. Both *BRCA* genes are passed on via autosomal dominant inheritance. This means that only one defective copy of the gene is required for the gene to be expressed. An individual with a parent carrying the mutated *BRCA1* gene has a one in two chance of inheriting the gene themselves. See **Figure 6.1** for diagrammatic representation of autosomal inheritance.

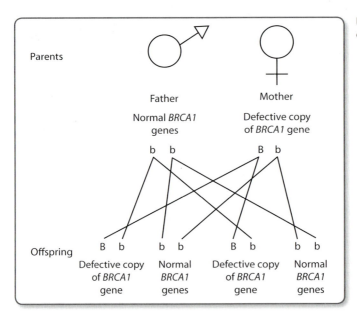

Figure 6.1 Autosomal dominant inheritance.

Families that carry either *BRCA1* or *BRCA2* mutations have a high incidence of breast and ovarian cancers (particularly of early onset), with individuals with the defective genes having an estimated 80% lifetime risk of breast cancer and up to a 40% lifetime risk of ovarian cancer.

6. D Robertsonian translocation

Familial Down's syndrome refers to trisomy 21 that occurs following a Robertsonian translocation. These translocations only occur in humans at chromosomes 13, 14, 15, 21 and 22. These chromosomes are acrocentric, i.e. they have very short arms. This form of translocation occurs when there is fusion of one acrocentric chromosome onto another acrocentric chromosome, so that their long arms become fused, with the loss of the insignificant genetic material found in the short arms. This may result in either a balanced Robertsonian translocation, whereby there is no overall loss or excess of chromosomal material, or an unbalanced translocation. In the latter there may be an extra copy of one of the chromosomes, i.e. a trisomy or a monosomy. Down's syndrome caused by a Robertsonian translocation is usually caused by the inheritance of two normal copies of chromosome 21 (one from each parent) and the inheritance of a balanced translocation chromosome from one parent. This translocation chromosome, typically chromosome 14, has a copy of chromosome 21 fused to its long arm, leading to trisomy 21. Couples where one partner carries such a translocation chromosome have around a 10% chance of each of their pregnancies being affected by Down's syndrome.

7. A Alpha-thalassaemia with deletion of 4 α-globin genes

Alpha-thalassaemia is an autosomal recessive condition associated with deletions in genes responsible for the production of α-globin chains. This couple both have α-thalassaemia trait, which means they each have either 2α-globin gene deletions on the same chromosomes or two chromosomes each with an α-globin gene deletion. Severity of α-thalassaemia is largely dependent on the number of α-globin genes affected. Individuals with the α-thalassaemia trait are usually minimally affected other than a mild anaemia. However, in fetuses with deletions in all of the 4α-globin chains there is a complete absence of α-globin production. In early fetal life, embryonic globin and gamma chains form functional units. At later gestations there is formation of haemoglobin Bart's (excess gamma chains which form tetramers) which has a high affinity for oxygen and therefore little oxygen delivery capacity. Hydrops fetalis is seen in fetuses with this profound absence of α-globin. Previously thought to be fatal, some fetuses may now survive with intrauterine transfusion.

Chapter 7

Physiology

Questions

For each question, select the single best answer from the five options listed.

1. A 32-year-old primiparous woman suffers a massive antepartum haemorrhage and undergoes an emergency caesarean section. During the caesarean section she suffers a massive obstetric haemorrhage and requires transfusion of blood and clotting factors. As a result, she develops disseminated intravascular coagulopathy.

   Which of the following laboratory results would be expected in this condition?

   A   Decreased activated partial thromboplastin time
   B   Increased factor VII levels
   C   Increased fibrinogen
   D   Increased soluble fibrin
   E   Thrombocytopaenia

2. A 23-year-old woman develops a fever, and has offensive vaginal discharge and abdominal pain. You are concerned that she is septic and wish to administer intravenous antibiotics. Prior to administration you wish to calculate her estimated glomerular filtration rate (eGFR) in order to dose her antibiotic therapy appropriately.

   Which of the following factors is included when calculating eGFR?

   A   Creatinine
   B   Diabetic status
   C   Height
   D   Medication
   E   Weight

3. A 25-year-old primiparous woman attends the antenatal clinic for a routine check at 28 weeks' gestation. Her urine dipstick shows glucose 2+. On questioning, she has just eaten a doughnut.

   Which of the following describes the sequential handling of glucose by the kidney?

   A   Filtered, reabsorbed and secreted
   B   Filtered, reabsorbed and not secreted
   C   Filtered, secreted, but not reabsorbed
   D   Filtered and neither secreted or reabsorbed
   E   Unfiltered, secreted

4. A 37-year-old woman attends her general practitioner for contraceptive advice. She smokes 10 cigarettes a day and has two children. She is keen to try the progesterone-only pill and asks you how it works.

    Which is the most appropriate answer?

    A   Creates a hostile environment for fertilisation to occur
    B   Creates an inflammatory reaction
    C   Inhibits ovulation
    D   Prevents implantation
    E   Thickens cervical mucus

5. A 72-year-old woman undergoes a total abdominal hysterectomy. She has chronic obstructive pulmonary disease. Postoperatively, she is difficult to extubate and has a prolonged stay on the intensive care unit.

    Which of the following is the most important direct stimulus to respiration?

    A   Decreased arterial pH
    B   Decreased arterial pO_2
    C   Decreased arterial pCO_2
    D   Increased H^+ concentration of the cerebrospinal fluid
    E   Increased pCO_2 of the cerebrospinal fluid

6. A 27-year-old woman attends antenatal clinic at 32 weeks' gestation complaining of gradual increasing shortness of breath through pregnancy. Although you feel it is important to exclude serious pathology, you are aware that this could be a normal symptom of advancing pregnancy.

    Which of the following contributors to lung volume and capacity occurs in normal pregnancy?

    A   Chest compliance increases
    B   Expiratory reserve volume increases
    C   Residual volume decreases
    D   Tidal volume decreases by up to 40%
    E   Vital capacity decreases

7. A 32-year-old woman is readmitted to the postnatal ward 10 days after an emergency caesarean section with a painful, swollen calf. Her observations are stable. Her body mass index is 37 kg/m². You want to rule out a deep vein thrombosis.

    Which of the following clotting factors are increased in normal pregnancy?

    A   Factor VII
    B   Factors VII and VII
    C   Factors VII, VIII and X
    D   Factors VII, VIII, X and XI
    E   Factors VII, VIII, X, XI and XIII

8. With regards to the cardiac cycle, what is the definition of stroke volume?

    A   Stroke volume = cardiac output / body surface area
    B   Stroke volume = end diastolic volume – end systolic volume
    C   Stroke volume = end systolic volume – end diastolic volume
    D   Stroke volume = end systolic volume + end diastolic volume
    E   Stroke volume = end diastolic volume + end systolic volume

9. A 2-week-old neonate is admitted to hospital with failure to thrive, tachypnoea and difficulty feeding. He is thought to have a circulatory defect.

Administration of prostaglandin antagonists soon after birth can be used to therapeutically close which patent structure of fetal origin?

    A   Ductus arteriosus
    B   Ductus venosus
    C   Foramen ovale
    D   Fossa ovalis
    E   Ligamentum venosum

10. A 67-year-old woman is admitted to hospital with frequency of urination and extreme thirst. Blood tests reveal deranged urea and electrolytes. The provisional diagnosis is diabetes insipidus.

Which hormone acts in the nephron, to increase the permeability of the collecting ducts to water?

    A   Aldosterone
    B   Angiotensin
    C   Atrial natriuretic peptide
    D   Parathyroid hormone
    E   Vasopressin

11. A 22-year-old woman is breastfeeding an hour after delivery. During lactation the 'let-down' reflex is stimulated by the action of which hormone?

    A   Human placental lactogen
    B   Oestrogen
    C   Oxytocin
    D   Prolactin
    E   Progesterone

12. A 27-year-old woman is being treated for primary infertility. A pelvic ultrasound shows multiple small ovarian follicles present in both ovaries. She is having ultrasound tracking of her ovaries as she has an irregular cycle.

What is the approximate size of the dominant ovarian follicle at the time of ovulation?

    A   1–2 mm
    B   5 mm

C   20 mm
D   30–40 mm
E   50 mm

13. A 33-year-old woman attends antenatal clinic at 33 weeks' gestation complaining of shortness of breath.

   Which of the following causes a shift of oxygen dissociation to the left?

   A   Decreased haemoglobin
   B   Decreased 2,3-diphosphoglycerate
   C   Increased acidity
   D   Increased carbon dioxide
   E   Increased temperature

14. Which of the following substances is unable to bind with fetal haemoglobin?

   A   2,3-diphosphoglycerate
   B   Carbon dioxide
   C   Carbon monoxide
   D   Nitrous oxide
   E   Oxygen

15. A 72-year-old woman is undergoing lung function tests prior to abdominal surgery.

   Which of the following gives the correct lung volume equation?

   A   Functional residual capacity = residual volume + tidal volume
   B   Inspiratory capacity = tidal volume + expiratory reserve volume
   C   Inspiratory capacity = inspiratory reserve volume – tidal volume
   D   Total lung capacity = inspiratory capacity + residual volume
   E   Vital capacity = inspiratory capacity + expiratory reserve volume

Answers

1. E Thrombocytopaenia

Disseminated intravascular coagulopathy (DIC) is a condition where generalised and widespread pathological activation of the clotting system occurs. There is clotting within the microvasculature which causes consumption of coagulation products. Pathological changes include inflammatory activation, suppression of anticoagulation and inhibition of fibrinolysis. The obstruction of the microvascular vessels can cause disruption of blood flow to major organs, potentially leading to multiorgan failure.

DIC usually occurs as a result of activation of the intrinsic coagulation pathway. There are usually increased levels of soluble fibrin. Diagnosis is by blood tests which usually reveal:

- Thrombocytopaenia
- Prolonged activated partial thromboplastin time
- Low fibrinogen
- Increased fibrinogen degradation products

Treatment is via reversal of the underlying cause. Fresh frozen plasma may be given as well as platelets depending on the degree of thrombocytopaenia.

2. A Creatinine

Estimated glomerular filtration rate is used as a marker of renal function and used in clinical practice, e.g. for calculations of renal function in the use of nephrotoxic drugs. It is often calculated using the modification of diet in renal disease (MDRD) equation which takes into account the age, creatinine levels, gender and ethnic group. Weight, height, comorbidities and medication are not used in this formula. It must be remembered that estimated glomerular filtration rate (eGFR) is still an estimate and may be inaccurate in certain circumstances, for instance with malnourished patients and amputees. It should not be used in children or pregnant women. For Afro-Caribbean patients, the eGFR may be 21% higher than estimated. Normal GFR is > 90 mL/min / 1.73 m^2.

3. B Filtered, reabsorbed and not secreted

In the normally-functioning kidneys, glucose is filtered, reabsorbed via secondary active transport and is generally not secreted in the urine. Virtually all glucose is reabsorbed in the apical region of proximal convoluted tubule of the kidney via Na/glucose transporters and also by glucose transporters (GLUTs). When the level of plasma glucose exceeds the filtering capacity of the kidneys, the amount of glucose excreted in the urine increases. The renal threshold for glucose, that is the amount of plasma glucose that the kidneys are able to filter without it being excreted in large amounts in the urine, is around 200 mg/dL. Glycosuria may be suggestive of diabetes mellitus and requires further investigation.

4. E Thickens cervical mucus

If taken appropriately, the progesterone-only pill (POP) is approximately 99% effective. Its main mechanism of action is by thickening the cervical secretions. It also thins the endometrium and makes the embryo less likely to implant. The POP is only effective if taken at the same time every day or within a 3-hour window. This is due to the mechanism of action of the POP which loses efficacy if there is a delay in taking it. The combined oral contraceptive pill works by inhibiting ovulation. The intrauterine contraceptive device provides a hostile environment and prevents implantation. It may also cause an inflammatory reaction. The copper of the copper coil also prevents the sperm from entering the uterus.

5. D Increased H⁺ concentration of the cerebrospinal fluid

The main stimulus to the respiratory centre comes from the chemoreceptors. These are central and peripheral. The central chemoreceptors are found on the surface of the upper medulla. Peripheral chemoreceptors are around the aortic arch, innervated by the vagus nerve, and in the carotid body, innervated by the glossopharyngeal nerve. The central chemoreceptors are only sensitive to changes in the pH. The carotid body receptors are sensitive to changes in pO_2. Both the carotid body and aortic arch receptors are sensitive to changes in pCO_2 and pH. Variations in CO_2 are altered via a change in ventilation. A rise in CO_2 leads to an increase in ventilation and hypoxia increases the respiratory centre sensitivity to CO_2. The response to hypoxia is less marked than the response to CO_2. The response to respiration as a result of acidosis is reduced because of the production of deoxygenated haemoglobin which acts as a buffer.

6. C Residual volume decreases

Table 7.1 summarises the change in lung function tests that occur as a result of pregnancy.

Table 7.1 Changes in respiratory system during pregnancy		
Increase	**Decrease**	**No change**
Tidal volume – up to 40%	Total lung capacity	Vital capacity
	Residual volume	Respiratory rate
	Expiratory reserve volume – approximately 200 mL	Lung compliance
	Inspiratory reserve volume	FEV1/PEFR
	Chest compliance	
	Airway resistance	

FEV1, forced expiratory volume in 1 second; PEFR, peak expiratory flow rate.

7. C Factors VII, VIII and X

In order to prepare the body to achieve rapid haemostasis after delivery, pregnancy is essentially a hypercoagulant state. As a consequence there is an increase in the majority of clotting factors during pregnancy, in particular factors VII, VIII and X. Factors XI and XIII do not change significantly during pregnancy.

Fibrinogen and erythrocyte sedimentation ratio may be doubled by term. There is an increase in antithrombin III and fibrinogen degradation products. The inhibition of fibrinolysis is partly mediated through placental plasminogen activator inhibitor (PAI2). PAI2 is a coagulation factor that is produced by the placenta and is only detectable in the blood during pregnancy. It activates tissue plasminogen activator and urokinase and is found in monocytes and macrophages.

The procoagulant state of pregnancy is one of the processes in place to prevent excess bleeding after delivery. Other mechanisms include uterine contraction and the development of a fibrin mesh which covers the placental site.

8. B Stroke volume = end diastolic volume – end systolic volume

The cardiac cycle is the repeated action of contraction and relaxation that leads to the pumping of blood from the heart and maintenance of circulation. Myocardial cells contract during electrical excitation and relax during repolarisation. During diastole the heart chambers relax and fill with blood. During systole, there is contraction of the ventricles and ejection of blood into the circulation. The atria contract together, with contraction of the ventricles occurring 0.1–0.2 seconds later.

Concerning the left side of the heart: at the beginning of ventricular systole, the mitral valve is open and the pressure in the left atrium is greater than that in the ventricle. As the pressure in the left atrium builds up, the mitral valve closes. Stroke volume is the calculated by subtracting the end systolic volume from the end diastolic volume. This is actually around 60–70% of blood left in the ventricles at the end of diastole. Stroke volume usually refers to the left ventricle, although it can be applied to both. Both ventricles have an equivalent stroke volume, which in the average sized adult is approximately 70 mL.

9. A Ductus arteriosus

The ductus arteriosus is one of the three circulatory shunts that exist in the fetal circulation. It is the fetal connection between the pulmonary artery and the aorta, allowing oxygenated fetal blood to be carried from the right ventricle and around the body, largely bypassing the lungs. It remains open throughout the fetal period due to high levels of vasodilating prostaglandins and also due to the low oxygen tension associated with the non-functioning pulmonary circulatory system. The ductus arteriosus usually closes permanently in the first few days of life as prostaglandin levels fall and as oxygen tensions dramatically rise after the first breath, leading to a rise in systemic circulatory pressure and fall in pressure of the previously high-resistance pulmonary circulation. A patent ductus arteriosus (PDA) is associated with prematurity and with other causes including maternal rubella infection during pregnancy. Children with a PDA may be asymptomatic, however young babies may present in the few weeks of life with tachypnoea, failure to thrive and difficulties with feeding. Prostaglandin antagonists such as non-steroidal anti-inflammatory drugs (NSAIDs) may be used to therapeutically close a PDA. Usage of NSAIDs can cause constriction of the fetal ductus arteriosus and hence all NSAIDs should be avoided in the third trimester of pregnancy.

10. E Vasopressin

Nephrons are the functional unit of the kidney and are responsible for the filtration of blood, excretion of waste products and the regulation of water balance. The collecting duct is the terminal part of the nephron and receives filtrate that has already passed through the glomerulus (the main functional filtration unit), the loop of Henle and the proximal and distal convoluted tubules. By the time the filtrate reaches the collecting duct it has already undergone a process of reabsorption of substances such as sodium chloride, water, bicarbonate, potassium and calcium. At the collecting duct vasopressin, also known as antidiuretic hormone, increases permeability to water, allowing for water molecules to be reabsorbed. Vasopressin enables the production of concentrated urine by acting on the aquaporins (water channels) of the collecting duct, allowing them to facilitate the passive reabsorption of water (**Figure 7.1**).

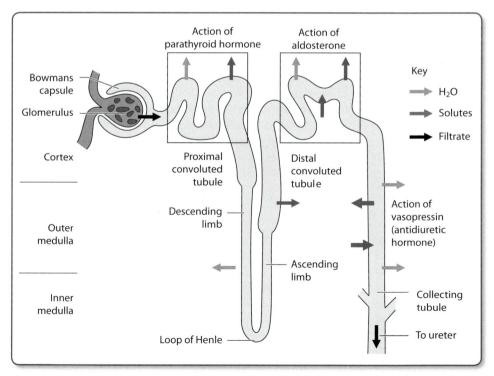

Figure 7.1 The nephron.

11. C Oxytocin

The 'let-down reflex', also known as the milk ejection reflex, describes the release of breast milk following the stimulus of suckling. The reflex is controlled by the action of the hormone oxytocin which is released from the hypothalamus in response to suckling, and causes contraction of the myoepithelial cells of the milk ducts, subsequently leading to milk ejection. Conditioning of this reflex occurs naturally to the extent that milk ejection may occur in lactating women in response to stimuli such as the sound of crying babies. Actual production of milk is largely under the control of prolactin which is released from the anterior pituitary gland in increasing amounts from early pregnancy.

12. C 20 mm

The dominant ovarian follicle grows considerably throughout folliculogenesis and by the time of ovulation has reached approximately 20 mm in size. It reaches the surface of the ovary and its release is due to necrobiosis of the overlying tissue. The rise in basal body temperature is thought to be due to the thermogenic effect of progesterone on the brain. The actual process of follicular rupture takes a few minutes. Mittelschmerz is the midcycle lower abdominal pain experienced by almost 1 in 4 women. This is thought to be caused by the release of follicular fluid leading to peritoneal irritation.

13. B Decreased 2,3-diphosphoglycerate

The oxygen dissociation curve is a graph which demonstrates the percentage saturation of haemoglobin at different partial pressures of oxygen. At higher partial pressures of oxygen, the haemoglobin binds with oxygen to form oxyhaemoglobin.

Each molecule of haemoglobin can bind with four molecules of oxygen. The sigmoid shape of the curve is a result of 'cooperation' between the oxygen binding site, i.e.

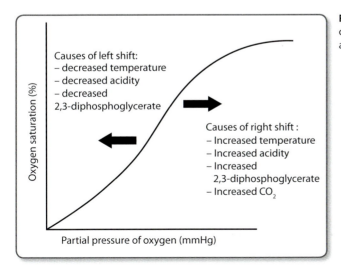

Figure 7.2 Oxygen dissociation curve with factors causing left and right shift.

occupancy of one of the binding sites makes it easier for the second to bind and the same with the third and fourth.

A right shift in the oxygen dissociation curve indicates a reduced oxygen affinity (**Figure 7.2**). This occurs when there is an increase in:

- Temperature
- Acidity
- 2,3-diphosphoglycerate
- Carbon dioxide

14. A 2,3-diphosphoglycerate

The oxygen dissociation curve for fetal haemoglobin (HbF) is a sigmoid shape. HbF consists of two α chains and two γ chains. HbF has a higher affinity for oxygen and there is therefore a left shift in the fetal oxygen dissociation curve. The reason for this shift is the reduced binding of 2,3-diphosphoglyceric acid (2,3-DPG). 2,3-DPG has a higher affinity for the β chains in the adult haemoglobin (HbA). This difference in binding capacity between HbA and HbF ensures that HbF has a greater affinity for oxygen than HbA. The P50 is defined as the partial pressure of oxygen at which the oxygen-carrying protein is 50% saturated and this is lower in HbF due to the reduced sensitivity of 2,3-DPG (**Figure 7.3**).

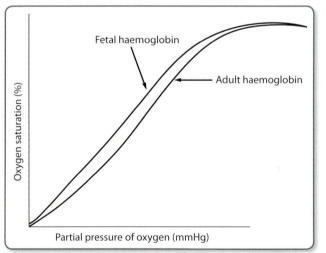

Figure 7.3 Fetal-maternal oxygen dissociation curves.

15. E Vital capacity = inspiratory capacity + expiratory reserve volume

Vital capacity describes the maximum volume of air that a person can exhale after maximum inspiration. It is therefore the combination of inspiratory capacity and the expiratory reserve volume. The inspiratory capacity is the combination of inspiratory reserve volume plus the tidal volume and is approximately 2.4 L in a female adult. The expiratory reserve volume is determined by the functional residual volume minus the residual volume. Vital capacity may be measured by spirometry and forms one element of a basic lung function test.

Chapter 8

Biophysics

Questions

For each question, select the single best answer from the five options listed.

1. Which of the following describes the mode used in creating standard grey scale ultrasound images?

    A   A-mode
    B   B-mode
    C   Doppler mode
    D   M-mode
    E   None of above

2. Which of the following is a recognised parameter used in fetal biophysical profiling?

    A   Abdominal circumference
    B   Amniotic fluid index
    C   Biparietal diameter
    D   Head circumference
    E   Femur length

3. Which of the following modalities uses an ionising form of radiation?

    A   Electrocautery
    B   Laser
    C   Magnetic resonance imaging
    D   Ultrasound
    E   X-ray

4. The standard chest X-ray is equivalent to what duration of natural background radiation:

    A   3 days
    B   20 days
    C   2 months
    D   1 year
    E   3 years

5. At what crown–rump length would you first expect to see a fetal heart beat using transvaginal ultrasonography?

    A   >2 mm
    B   >3 mm
    C   >4 mm
    D   >5 mm
    E   >6 mm

6. A 68-year-old woman developed left-sided chest pain a day after she has had total abdominal hysterectomy and bilateral-salpingo-oophorectomy. A 12-lead electrocardiogram is performed and is suggestive of an anterior ST elevation myocardial infarction.

    Which of the following leads would be most likely to show ST elevation in this patient?

    A   I, aVL, V_5–V_6
    B   I, II and III
    C   II, III and aVF
    D V_1–V_4
    E   All of the above

7. Which of the following is a late side-effect of radiotherapy?

    A   Fatigue
    B   Lymphoedema
    C   Mouth ulcers
    D   Nausea
    E   Oedema

8. Which of the following best describes acoustic impedance?

    A   It is an estimate of mean velocity of flow within a vessel
    B   It is the apparent bending of waves
    C   It is the opposition to the passage of sound waves and is a function of density and elasticity
    D   It is when reflected waves from a moving interface undergo a frequency shift
    E   It is the angle at which the wave is incident on the surface equals the angle of reflection

9. A dual energy X-ray absorptiometry (DEXA) scan is used to assess bone mineral density in possible cases of osteoporosis.

    What type and how many beams of X-ray are used with a DEXA scan?

    A   One high dose X-ray beam
    B   One low dose X-ray beam
    C   Two high dose X-ray beams
    D   Two low dose X-ray beams
    E   Three medium dose X-ray beams

10. An 80-year-old woman attends pre-assessment clinic prior to a vaginal wall repair. She is found to have first-degree heart block on electrocardiogram.

   An extended P-R interval in an electrocardiogram may represent heart block. What is the normal P-R interval?

   A   0–40 ms
   B   40–120 ms
   C   80–400 ms
   D   120–200 ms
   E   160–240 ms

11. A woman undergoes a Caesarean section where diathermy is used for haemostasis. During electrosurgery, at what temperature does coagulation take place?

   A   25°C
   B   70°C
   C   120°C
   D   200°C
   E   400°C

12. Radiotherapy commonly uses ionising radiation to damage target DNA. What are the units used to measure absorbed radiotherapy dose?

   A   Hertz
   B   Grays
   C   Sievert
   D   Tesla
   E   Weber

13. Diathermy is a frequently used modality in surgery. What is the name of the property of diathermy that causes extreme drying to the tissue?

   A   Coagulation
   B   Conduction
   C   Cutting
   D   Desiccation
   E   Fulguration

Answers

1. B B-mode

A-mode is the simplest form of ultrasound and is now rarely used. It creates wave spikes as the ultrasound comes into contact with various tissues. The distance between the spikes can be measured. The A in A-mode refers to the amplitude of the ultrasound used. B-mode, or brightness mode, is widely used in ultrasound to create two-dimensional greyscale images obtained from a linear array of transducers, which simultaneously scan a tissue plane. M-mode incorporates movement with successive A- or B-mode images. Doppler mode is used to assess movement and is the mode used for looking at blood flow. There are various different types of Doppler used including pulsed wave, continuous and colour.

2. B Amniotic fluid index

Biophysical profiling provides a means of formally assessing fetal well-being.

This may be indicated in the context of reduced fetal movements or growth restriction. There are five biophysical variables which are assessed in biophysical profiling. Fetal tone, breathing, movement and heart rate are recorded, alongside an assessment of the amniotic fluid index. The assessment of the fetal heart rate is described as a non-stress test. A score is given for each variable and the total can then guide further management. The fetal head circumference, abdominal circumference, femur length and biparietal diameter are parameters used to assess fetal growth and are not part of biophysical profiling.

3. E X-ray

High energy forms of radiation capable of separating an electron from an atom are described as 'ionising'. Forms of ionising radiation can have therapeutic properties, but require close regulation to prevent excessive exposure. **Table 8.1** lists sources of ionising and non-ionising radiation.

Table 8.1 Examples of ionising and non-ionising radiation	
Ionising radiation	**Non-ionising radiation**
X-ray	Electrocautery
Radiotherapy	Laser
Positron emission tomography	MRI
Radionucleotides, e.g. barium swallow	Ultrasound
	Microwaves
	Diathermy

4. A 3 days

Radiation dosage is measured in millisieverts (mSv) and is often referred to as the effective dose. Exposure to radiation can also be described in terms of the equivalent duration of natural background radiation associated with the exposure. For different imaging modalities, **Table 8.2** gives the time it would take to receive an equivalent radiation does from natural background radiation dose.

Table 8.2 Imaging modalities with equivalent natural background radiation	
Modality	**Equivalent time period from natural background radiation**
Chest X-ray	3 days
CT of abdomen	4.5
Lumbar spine X-ray	7 months
Intravenous urogram	14 months

5. A >2 mm

Fetal heart action should be evident when the crown–rump length (CRL) is >2 mm.

In 5–10% of embryos there will be no fetal heart action visible until > 4 mm. When using ultrasound to diagnose the viability of a pregnancy, a CRL of ≥7 mm and absence of fetal heart action suggests a non-viable pregnancy. In these cases a further scan may be indicated after an interval of at least 1 week.

National Institute for Health and Clinical Excellence. Ectopic pregnancy and miscarriage: diagnosis and initial management. Clinical Guideline CG154. London: NICE, 2012

6. D V_1–V_4

Varying electrode placement allows the electrocardiogram to create a pictorial representation of electrical activity in the heart. It is possible to localise pathological changes in the heart's conduction pathways. Leads V_1–V_4 detect electrical activity in the anterior part of the heart along the horizontal plane. Therefore, when there is a considerable change in the heart conduction pathways as a consequence of an anterior myocardial infarction we may expect to see ST wave elevation in these leads. An inferior ST elevation myocardial infarction (STEMI) would be represented as ST wave elevation in leads II, III and aVF. Electrical activity in the lateral aspect of the heart is monitored by V_5 and V_6, as well by as leads I and aVL. A lateral STEMI is likely to be seen as ST elevation in leads I, aVL and V_5 to V_6.

7. B Lymphoedema

Radiotherapy is a form of ionising radiation that is widely used in the treatment of cancers, but may also be used for a variety of non-malignant conditions. Radiotherapy is effective in damaging the cellular DNA, thus causing cellular death.

The ionising radiation is targeted at localised areas to avoid generalised exposure to its effects. Like any intervention, radiotherapy has side effects which can be classified to acute or late (**Table 8.3**). Lymphoedema is one such late side effect and typically occurs following pelvic and breast radiotherapy.

Table 8.3 Side-effects of radiotherapy	
Acute	**Late**
Oedema	Lymphoedema
Gastrointestinal symptoms: nausea, vomiting, diarrhoea, abdominal pain	Hair loss
Fatigue	Development of further cancers
Epithelial surface damage, e.g. mouth ulcers	Tissue fibrosis
	Infertility

8. C It is the opposition to the passage of sound waves and is a function of density and elasticity

Acoustic impedance is a term used in the description of ultrasound behaviour within a tissue. It represents the opposition to the passage of sound waves and is a function of density and elasticity. Refraction is the change in direction of the wave as a result in change of speed. Diffraction describes the bending of waves as a result of interaction with obstacles. Reflected waves from a moving object undergoing a frequency shift is the Doppler effect. Colour Doppler provides an estimate of mean velocity of flow within a vessel.

9. D Two low dose X-ray beams

Dual energy X-ray absorptiometry (DEXA) scans provide a measure of bone mineral density (BMD). The use of two low-dose (1/10th of a standard chest X-ray) beams at the spine and hip aids determination of the BMD compared with control groups.

The T-score is used in adults and is calculated by comparing the patient's BMD with that of a young healthy adult; it is matched for gender and ethnic group (**Table 8.4**).

Table 8.4 T-score values	
Between +1 and −1 SD	Normal
Between −1 and −2.5 SD	Osteopenia
Below −2.5 SD	Osteoporosis

The Z-score is similar to the T-score, except it also matches for the patient's age, gender and ethnic group.

10. D 120–200 ms

The P-R interval represents the conduction through the AV node and is measured from the onset of the P wave to the beginning of the QRS complex.

The normal time for the P-R interval is 120–200 ms (3–5 small squares on standard ECG paper).

An extended P-R interval may represent heart block, of which there are different degrees:

- First-degree heart block is represented by a consistent P-R interval of more than 200 ms
- Second degree, Mobitz Type-1 block is also known as Wenckebach phenomenon, and is characterised by a progressive prolongation of the P-R interval, followed by a non-conducted P wave
- Second degree, Mobitz Type-2 block is characterised by non-conducted P waves without the progressive prolongation seen in Mobitz type 1 block
- Third degree (complete) heart block is typified by complete absence of conduction of the signal generated from the SA node in the atrium to the ventricles. The ECG reveals two independent rhythms; one represented by the P-waves, and a second represented by the QRS complexes

11. B 70°C

During electrosurgery, tissues undergo different changes at different temperatures achieved, which is important for optimising surgical technique.

Coagulation occurs at approximately 70°C, desiccation occurs at 90°C and carbonisation occurs at 200°C. Monopolar involves high density current through a small contact area. The current will flow from the generator to the patient and then back to the generator through the return electrode (diathermy pad). An earth pad is required on the patient. Cutting and coagulation is possible when using monopolar energy. Cutting mode uses a continuous waveform of low voltage, whereas coagulation uses intermittent waveforms, allowing the tissue to cool between bursts of high voltage energy. Bipolar instruments have two electrodes (one active and one return electrode) on one instrument through which the current passes.

12. B Grays

The international system of units (SI) is the widely recognised system for measuring different modalities.

Units	Modality
Hertz (Hz)	Frequency
Tesla (T)	Magnetic field strength
Sievert (Sv)	Equivalent dose (of ionising radiation)
Gray (Gy)	Absorbed dose (of ionising radiation)

Radiotherapy uses ionising radiation to target malignancy by damaging DNA. This is caused by free radicals created when intracellular water molecules are ionised.

Internal beam therapies, including radioisotopes are delivered by injection to irradiate the whole body. Alternatively, brachytherapy is delivered as a sealed source close to the diseased tissue, providing less collateral damage to healthy tissue.

Adjunctive radiotherapy is given after surgical removal and aims to reduce the risk of recurrence. Neo-adjunctive therapy is delivered before surgery and aims to reduce the size of a tumour to improve surgical outcome.

13. D Desiccation

Coagulation is the process of changing blood from a liquid to a gel, potentially resulting in haemostasis. Desiccation is characterised by extreme drying of affected tissue, and fulguration destroys tissue using high frequency electrical current through a thin electrode.

Chapter 9

Clinical management

Questions

For each question, select the single best answer from the five options listed.

1. A 22-year-old patient, who is 35 weeks pregnant, presents to the hospital complaining of heavy painless bleeding. She is pale, has a pulse rate of 140 beats per minute, and a blood pressure of 70/40 mmHg. Her abdomen is soft and non-tender.

   What is the most likely diagnosis?

   A   Concealed abruption
   B   Placenta praevia
   C   Premature labour
   D   Revealed abruption
   E   Vasa praevia

2. A 40-year-old woman complains of heavy regular periods for 5 years. Ultrasound scan has revealed no abnormality. Her family is complete.

   What is the most appropriate first line treatment for this patient?

   A   Combined oral contraceptive pill
   B   Laparoscopic assisted vaginal hysterectomy
   C   Levonorgestrel-releasing intrauterine system
   D   Norethisterone tablet 5 mg three times daily from day 5–26 of menstrual cycle
   E   Tranexamic acid

3. A 35-year-old woman attends gynaecology outpatient department with an incidental ultrasound finding of a 4 cm simple ovarian cyst.

   What is the most appropriate plan of management?

   A   Consider further imaging (i.e. MRI)
   B   Laparoscopic cystectomy
   C   Reassure and discharge
   D   Serum CA-125 test
   E   Yearly ultrasound follow-up

4. A 22-year-old woman with a past history of chlamydia attends the emergency department complaining of severe abdominal pain. She has mild vaginal bleeding. Her pulse rate is 120 beats per minute, with a blood pressure of 60/40 mmHg and she has a distended tender abdomen.

   What is the most likely diagnosis?

   A   Acute appendicitis
   B   Complete miscarriage
   C   Ruptured ectopic pregnancy
   D   Threatened miscarriage
   E   Urinary tract infection

5. You are asked to review a 20-year-old woman in the Emergency Department. She has a positive pregnancy test, and is unsure of her last menstrual period. On examination, her pulse is 70 beats per minute and her blood pressure is 110/70 mmHg. Her abdomen is soft and non-tender. Speculum examination reveals a closed cervix and mild bleeding.

   What is the most appropriate plan of management?

   A   Admit the patient and arrange an evacuation of retained products of conception
   B   Admit the patient for a laparoscopy as an ectopic pregnancy cannot be excluded
   C   Admit the patient for hourly observations
   D   Arrange the next available ultrasound scan as an outpatient
   E   Discharge the patient with the diagnosis of complete miscarriage

6. A 30-year-old patient, who is hypertensive and obese with a body mass index of 38 kg/m², requests contraception. She has had two previous caesarean sections.

   What is the most effective and safest form of contraception for her?

   A   Laparoscopic sterilisation
   B   Combined oral contraceptive pill
   C   Subdermal implant
   D   Barrier contraception
   E   Intrauterine device

7. A 44-year-old is 28 weeks pregnant following ovum donation. She presents with headache and reports seeing 'flashing lights'. Her blood pressure is 172/112 mmHg and her pulse rate is 78 beats per minute. Urine dipstick shows protein +++, leucocytes trace, nitrites negative, blood trace.

   Which is the most appropriate immediate management for this patient?

   A   Request an urgent scan for fetal growth
   B   Administer antihypertensives to lower her blood pressure
   C   Administer ramipril
   D   Avoid steroid injections as it will worsen her blood pressure
   E   Immediate delivery of the baby by category one caesarean section

8. The risk of malignancy index (RMI) is used to score the risk of ovarian cancer in women.

   Which of the following is correct with regards to the basis of its calculation?

   A   Classification of post-menopausal is a woman who has had no periods for 2 years or over age of 51 years
   B   Premenopausal status is scored as 3
   C   Serum CA-125 levels are measured on a scale of 1 to 10
   D   Ultrasound scan must show a cyst of at least 10 cm in size
   E   Ultrasound score × menopausal status × CA-125

9. A 27-year-old woman attends the antenatal clinic at 14 weeks' gestation in her third pregnancy. She had a deep vein thrombosis from when she broke her leg during a skiing trip at age 20 years. Her thrombophilia screen outside of pregnancy was negative. She has no family history of venous thromboembolism.

   Which of the following is the most appropriate action?

   A   Aspirin 150 mg from conception to 36 weeks' gestation
   B   Low-molecular weight heparin therapy immediately
   C   Low-molecular weight heparin therapy from 24 weeks' gestation until onset of labour
   D   Low-molecular weight heparin therapy for 6 weeks postnatally
   E   Referral to haematology for repeat thrombophilia screen now she is pregnant

10. A 47-year-old premenopausal woman undergoes a hysteroscopy for investigation of severe menorrhagia. Histology of the endometrial biopsy shows simple hyperplasia.

    What would be the most appropriate recommendation?

    A   Commence hormone replacement therapy
    B   Hysterectomy
    C   Insertion of a levonorgestrel-releasing intrauterine system
    D   Ultrasound scan in 6 months
    E   No treatment is required

11. A 32-year-old primiparous woman is in labour. Labour was induced at 40 + 12 weeks for post-dates and oxytocin augmentation has been used. Following delivery of the fetal head the midwife is unable to deliver the body using gentle traction. She suspects there is 'shoulder dystocia' and the emergency buzzer is pulled.

    Which of the following is the most appropriate first line measure to be taken in order to deliver the baby?

    A   Episiotomy
    B   Fundal pressure
    C   McRoberts' manoeuvre
    D   Symphysiotomy
    E   Zavanelli manoeuvre

12. A 28-year-old primiparous woman is 24 weeks pregnant. She presents to the Maternity Day Unit with a history of reduced fetal movements over the last 18 hours. She is well and has no medical or obstetric history of note.

    What is the most appropriate means of assessing fetal well-being in this pregnancy?

    A   Auscultation of the fetal heart using a handheld Doppler device
    B   Biophysical profiling
    C   Cardiotocograph
    D   Completion of 24-hour kick chart
    E   Ultrasound scan

13. A 36-year-old nulliparous woman and her partner are seen in fertility clinic for the first time. They have been unsuccessfully trying to conceive for the last 15 months. At this initial appointment you arrange a series of routine investigations, including semen analysis for the male partner.

    What advice should you give with regard to the collection of his semen?

    A   There is no need for any abstinence from ejaculation prior to collection
    B   He should abstain from ejaculation 2–3 days prior to collection
    C   He should abstain from ejaculation for seven days prior to collection
    D   He should abstain from ejaculation for 14 days prior to collection
    E   He should provide his second ejaculate within a 24-hour period for collection

14. A 23-year-old nulliparous woman is seen in gynaecology out-patient clinic for the first time. She has been referred by her general practitioner with a 12-month history of heavy menstrual bleeding. She is keen for investigation and management of her symptoms.

    Which of the following is an appropriate first-line investigation of her menorrhagia?

    A   Coagulation screen
    B   Full blood count
    C   Hormone profile, including progesterone
    D   Serum ferritin
    E   Thyroid Function Test

15. A 33-year-old woman who has had two previous caesarean sections is seen in antenatal clinic in order to book and discuss her elective caesarean section. Her caesarean section is scheduled for 39 weeks' gestation. The hospital's laboratory will require a serum group and screen sample.

    When is it most appropriate to take this serum group and screen sample?

    A   At her antenatal booking appointment
    B   At 28 weeks' gestation

C Within 3 days of the planned caesarean section
D Within 5 days of the planned caesarean section
E Within 10 days of the planned caesarean section

16. A 39-year-old multiparous woman is seen in gynaecology out-patient clinic. She has suffered from heavy menstrual bleeding for several years and now seeks advice on how to improve her symptoms. A recent transvaginal ultrasound scan of her pelvis showed an anteverted uterus with two small 2 cm intramural fibroids, with no distortion of the uterine cavity seen. She is not keen to conceive in the future.

Which of the following is the most appropriate first line treatment to offer her?

A Endometrial ablation
B Levonorgestrel-releasing intrauterine system
C Mefenamic acid
D Tranexamic acid
E Vaginal hysterectomy

17. A 27-year-old multiparous woman presents to Maternity Triage at 26 weeks' gestation. She appears drowsy, is sweating and reports a headache, general tiredness and feeling cold. On questioning she gives a history of returning from a country where malaria is endemic 2 days ago. Her blood pressure is 102/68 mmHg, her pulse rate is 110 beats per minutes, her temperature 38.5°C and her respiratory rate is 24 breaths per minute. A blood film has been urgently requested to look for malaria parasites.

What percentage of parasitised red blood cells in a pregnant woman can indicate severe malaria?

A 2%
B 5%
C 15%
D 25%
E 50%

18. An unwell 32-year-old nulliparous woman is admitted to hospital at 32 weeks' gestation. She is drowsy, jaundiced with pyrexia of 38.8°C. She has recently returned from seeing family where malaria is endemic. Thick and thin malarial blood films indicate a severe *Plasmodium falciparum* parasitaemia.

What is the appropriate treatment for this patient?

A Artesunate
B Chloroquine
C Clindamycin
D Primaquine
E Quinine

19. A 22-year-old nulliparous woman is seen at 16 weeks' gestation in antenatal clinic. She has disclosed that she experienced female genital mutilation (FGM) as a child in her country of birth. She consents to have a vulval inspection and examination. It is evident that her clitoris and labia minora and labia majora have been completely excised; the vaginal orifice does not appear to be narrowed.

What type of FGM (according the WHO classification) has this woman been subjected to?

A   Type 1
B   Type 2
C   Type 3
D   Type 4
E   Type 5

Answers

1. B Placenta praevia

Placenta praevia is the partial or complete insertion of the placenta into the lower segment of the uterus. It is graded from I to IV, where grades I and II are classified as minor placenta praevia and grades III and IV as major placenta praevia. Minor placenta praevia is present when the placenta has inserted into the lower segment and is close to the cervical os. Major placenta praevia is present when the placenta lies over the cervical os. Women with placenta praevia may present with painless bleeding.

Vasa praevia is present when fetal vessels are found across the membranes over the internal os, below the presenting part. Bleeding from a placenta praevia carries risk to maternal life, whereas vasa praevia is associated with high levels of fetal morbidity and mortality due to fetal haemorrhage if immediate delivery is not undertaken.

2. C Levonorgestrel-releasing intrauterine system

Menorrhagia is a common problem, with one in three women describing their periods as 'heavy'. No obvious cause is found in approximately 50% of cases. The only routine investigation required is a full blood count (FBC), and other investigations, such as an ultrasound of the pelvis, should only be performed if indicated.

The use of a levonorgestrel-releasing intrauterine system (IUS) is currently the recommended first-line management option. With this form of IUS, the majority of women will have a reduction in their menstrual flow and in some women it may cause amenorrhoea. Second-line options include using tranexamic acid, non-steroidal anti-inflammatory drugs or the combined oral contraceptive pill.

3. C Reassure and discharge

The majority of ovarian cysts in premenopausal women are benign, with the risk of malignancy being 1–3 per 1000. Simple thin-walled cysts which are < 50 mm in diameter can be managed conservatively, and most of these are resolve within 3 months. A pelvic ultrasound is the most appropriate way of assessing an ovarian cyst, with the transvaginal route being more sensitive. See **Figure 9.1** for an ultrasound image of an ovarian cyst.

It is important to remember that CA-125 has an increased rate of false positives in premenopausal women. Its value may be raised in other conditions such as endometriosis, pelvic infection, endometriosis, and when a woman has fibroids. Therefore in the presence of a simple ovarian cyst taking a serum CA-125 level is not essential.

However, in women under 40 years of age with the ultrasound finding of a complex ovarian mass, tumour markers such as human chorionic gonadotropin, α-fetoprotein, and lactate should be measured to exclude germ cell tumours.

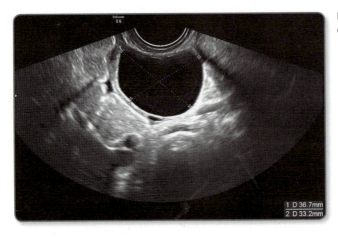

Figure 9.1 Ultrasound of ovarian cyst.

4. C Ruptured ectopic pregnancy

An ectopic pregnancy is one that is implanted outside the womb. It must be excluded in any woman who presents with abdominal or bowel symptoms with a positive pregnancy test. Previous pelvic inflammatory disease (PID) is a known risk factor. Other risk factors for ectopic pregnancy include previous pelvis or tubal surgery, endometriosis, assisted conception or a history of subfertility, smoking and the presence of an in situ intrauterine device.

The fallopian tube is the most common site of an ectopic pregnancy; however, they may also be abdominal, ovarian or cervical. The majority of ectopic pregnancies are in the ampullary segment of the fallopian tube.

The isthmic segment of the tube is narrower than the ampullary portion. As a consequence rupture occurs at earlier gestations with isthmic ectopic pregnancies. In contrast, rupture of the interstitial segment of the fallopian tube can occur at the relatively late gestation of 12–14 weeks.

5. D Arrange the next available ultrasound scan as an outpatient

Miscarriage is the most common complication of pregnancy. Threatened miscarriage is defined as uterine bleeding with a closed cervix. It can affect up to 25% of pregnancies. Clinical examination will reveal a soft, non-tender uterus.

An inevitable miscarriage is either complete or incomplete depending on whether all the pregnancy tissue has been expelled from the uterus or not. An incomplete miscarriage will present with ongoing bleeding, abdominal pain and an open cervix.

An early pregnancy assessment unit is an appropriate setting for referral of a haemodynamically stable patient in early pregnancy. Women need to know that until then an ectopic pregnancy cannot be excluded, and they must return earlier if they experience severe pain or become unwell.

6. C Subdermal implant

The subdermal implant is a progestogen-based contraception and is a form of long-acting reversible contraception. Once inserted, it is licensed for contraceptive use for 3 years. The main mode of action is inhibition of ovulation, but as it contains progestogen it also has progesterone contraception effects, including changes to cervical mucus and inhibition of normal endometrial development. Benefits include efficacy (pregnancy < 1 in 1000 over 3 years), length of efficacy and no user reliability. It obviously does not protect against sexually-transmitted infections and the major side effect of its use is irregular bleeding, which patients should be counselled about prior to insertion. Up to 20% of women will have no bleeding and up to half of women will experience irregular or infrequent bleeding.

7. B Administer antihypertensives to lower her blood pressure

This patient has pre-eclampsia, as indicated by her hypertension, proteinuria and symptoms. When a patient has severe pre-eclampsia it is important to keep her blood pressure $< 150/80$–100 mmHg. The first line antihypertensive is labetolol. Other options include methyldopa, hydralazine and nifedipine. Uncontrolled hypertension leads to both maternal and neonatal morbidity and mortality. If this patient's pre-eclampsia cannot be controlled she may require delivery. If delivery is thought to be likely in the next 7 days a course of steroids should be considered if the gestation is < 37 weeks.

8. E Ultrasound score × menopausal status × CA-125

The risk of malignancy index (RMI) uses three pre-surgical features in order to stratify an overall risk of having a malignant ovarian tumour.

It is calculated as RMI $= U \times M \times$ CA-125, where:

- U is the ultrasound result and gives a point for specific characteristics of the ovarian mass
- M is the menopausal status; being postmenopausal confers higher risk
- CA-125 is the serum level of the tumour marker, Cancer Antigen 125

National Institute for Health and Clinical Excellence. Ovarian Cancer: the Recognition and Initial Management of Ovarian Cancer. Clinical Guideline CG122. London: NICE, 2011.

9. D Low-molecular weight heparin therapy for 6 weeks postnatally

Any woman who has had only one thromboembolic event in the past, with no other known risk factors, still needs to be monitored closely during her pregnancy. A prophylactic dose of low molecular weight heparin is needed for 6 weeks after delivery. Factor V Leiden is the most common inherited thrombophilic disorder. The risk of thromboembolic events can be increased by approximately 30 times in individuals who are homozygous for the disease. This patient is most at risk of developing a thromboembolic event postnatally and the most appropriate course of action is to give low molecular weight heparin for 6 weeks postnatally.

10. C Insertion of a levonorgestrel-releasing intrauterine system

Endometrial hyperplasia is a premalignant condition and these patients are more likely to develop endometrial carcinoma. One important cause is unopposed oestrogens, therefore oestrogen-only hormone replacement therapy would be contraindicated in this case. An ultrasound in 6 months' time would not be the most appropriate management as it is not a diagnostic tool, and would only be of benefit to determine endometrial thickness. Use of progestogens helps to maintain a thin endometrium and prevent development of endometrial cancer.

11. C McRoberts' manoeuvre

Failure to deliver the fetal body, following delivery of the head, which requires the use of manoeuvres to release the impacted fetal shoulder is known as shoulder dystocia. This event is considered an obstetric emergency as the fetus can quickly become compromised and help should be called for immediately. The McRoberts' position requires flexion and abduction of both of the maternal hips. This manoeuvre is often sufficient to deliver the baby. Fundal pressure should not be applied at any point. Episiotomy may be performed to provide additional room for further internal manoeuvres but in itself does not aid delivery. The Zavanelli manoeuvre, which involves replacement of the baby's head prior to emergency caesarean section, is one of the last manoeuvres to resort to if all else has failed.

12. A Auscultation of the fetal heart using a handheld Doppler device

The perception of reduced fetal movement (RFM) is a common obstetric presentation. In the majority of presentations of RFM, fetal well-being is confirmed and the pregnancy goes on to have a successful outcome. Nevertheless, the sudden reduction in fetal movements or cessation of any movement perception must be taken seriously and is often reported by women who have had a stillbirth. Between 24 and 28 weeks' gestation the most appropriate investigation is auscultation of fetal heart using a handheld Doppler device. At this gestation there is neither role for cardiotocography (CTG) nor ultrasound assessment (unless there are other concerns regarding fetal growth). After 28 weeks a CTG is an appropriate method of assessing well-being. Prior to 24 weeks' gestation fetal well-being should be assessed using a handheld Doppler device (as for pregnancies of 24–28 weeks' gestation). The completion of a 24-hour kick chart following normal investigation of fetal well-being is not indicated at any gestation. Biophysical profiling is not indicated in low-risk pregnancies with RFM. Any woman who has further episodes of RFM should be advised to re-present to her care providers as soon as possible.

13. B He should abstain from ejaculation for 2–3 days prior to collection

Semen analysis is an essential investigation in the assessment and treatment of couples who are experiencing difficulty conceiving. Abstinence from ejaculation of two to three days prior to performing the semen analysis is recommended. Shorter periods of abstinence may result in production difficulties, whilst the longer periods of abstinence can lead to higher proportions of dead sperm and debris being present in the sample. In the presence of an abnormal result at semen analysis, a repeat sample should be arranged for three months' time, to give time for a full cycle of spermatozoa development.

14. B Full blood count

A full blood count is an essential investigation in the management of heavy menstrual bleeding and therefore is the most appropriate first-line investigation for this patient. Whilst a coagulation screen should be considered for a woman who has had menorrhagia since menarche or has a personal or family history which could suggest coagulation disorders, this is not a routine investigation. Serum ferritin should not typically be checked, nor should a female hormone profile be performed. It may be appropriate to do thyroid function tests if there are signs and symptoms of thyroid disease.

15. C Within 3 days of the planned caesarean section

A serum group and screen sample should be taken at every woman's antenatal booking appointment. A repeat sample should be taken at 28 weeks' gestation. As part of the work-up prior to their caesarean section each woman should have a fresh group and screen sample taken, so that any blood subsequently required for transfusion can be quickly cross-matched and made available. Any group and screen sample taken to facilitate blood transfusion in pregnancy should be no more than three days old. This relatively brief interval aims to ensure that the sample will reflect the patient's immune status, the presence of maternal red cell antibodies in pregnancy is relatively common. Consent should ideally always be obtained prior to any blood transfusion, although in some emergency situations this may not be possible.

16. B Levonorgestrel-releasing intrauterine system

If hormonal treatments are acceptable to a patient then the first line treatment is the levonorgestrel-releasing intrauterine system (LNG-IUS). Ideally the patient should be prepared to try the LNG-IUS for at least 12 months and should be made aware that it may cause irregular menstrual bleeding for the first 6 months after insertion. After the LNG-IUS it is appropriate to offer tranexamic acid in combination with mefenamic acid (if there is dysmenorrhoea).

Endometrial ablation may be appropriate in women who have severe menorrhagia, who do not want to conceive in the future, following consideration or trial of the above treatment options. Hysterectomy is not a first line treatment for menorrhagia.

17. A 2%

Malaria can be difficult to diagnose and may present as a flu-like illness. Pregnant women with parasitaemia of 2% or more are at risk of developing severe malaria which can manifest with respiratory distress, impaired consciousness or pulmonary oedema. Laboratory investigation may reveal severe anaemia, thrombocytopenia, hypoglycaemia and impaired renal function.

Malaria in pregnancy requires microscopic diagnosis. Rapid detection tests should be avoided in pregnancy as they may miss low parasitaemia and are relatively insensitive to *Plasmodium vivax* malaria. In a febrile patient, three negative malaria smears between 12 and 24 hours apart are needed to exclude diagnosis of malaria. Pregnant women with malaria should be admitted to hospital for treatment. Choloroquine is used for treatment of *Plasmodium vivax, Plasmodium ovale* or *Plasmodium malariae*. All infants born of mothers who had malaria in pregnancy should be screened as there is a risk of vertical transmission.

18. A Artesunate

Malaria in a pregnant woman should be treated as an emergency and treatment started as soon as possible. In uncomplicated malaria, fatality rates are low, approximately 0.1% for *Plasmodium falciparum*. In severe malaria, particularly in pregnancy, fatality rates are as high as 50%. Whilst admission to the ward is appropriate in mild cases, women with severe malaria should be admitted to the intensive care unit and the advice of the infectious diseases team sought. Severe *P. falciparum* malaria should be treated with intravenous artesunate, or if this not available then with intravenous quinine. Chloroquine is used in the treatment of *Plasmodium vivax, Plasmodium malariae* and *Plasmodium ovale*. Clindamycin may be used in combination with quinine in the treatment of uncomplicated *Plasmodium falciparum*.

Royal College of Obstetricians and Gynaecologists. The diagnosis and treatment of malaria in pregnancy. Green-top Guideline 54B. London: RCOG 2010.

19. B Type 2

Female genital mutilation (FGM) is both a form of child abuse and violation of human rights that is associated with significant physical and psychological morbidity in women and female children around the world. The World Health Organization (WHO) classification of FGM provides a useful means of determining severity on the basis of the anatomical structures that have been removed/mutilated.

Type 1	Partial or total removal of clitoris
Type 2	Partial or total removal of clitoris and labia minora (with or without excision of labia majora)
Type 3	Narrowing of the vaginal orifice, with creation of a covering seal by cutting and apositioning the labia minora and/or the labia majora, with or without excision of the clitoris
Type 4	All other harmful procedures to the female genitalia for non-medical purposes, including pricking, piercing, incising, scraping and cauterisation

Adapted from Annex 2: Note on the classification of female genital mutilation, Eliminating Female Genital Mutilation, An Interagency statement, World Health Organisation, 2008.

Chapter 10

Data interpretation

Questions

For each question, select the single best answer from the five options listed.

1. A fetal blood sample is performed on a 24-year-old primiparous woman at 7 cm dilatation due to a pathological cardiotocograph (CTG). The result shows a pH of 7.24.

    Based on this result, which is the most appropriate action?

    A   A repeat sample should be performed in 30 minutes
    B   It is a normal result and the patient should be reassured
    C   No further sample should be performed unless there is a terminal CTG
    D   Proceed for an urgent caesarean section
    E   The patient should be placed into left lateral position

2. An 18-year-old pregnant woman attends antenatal clinic at 32 weeks' gestation. Her urine sample reveals leucocytes 2+. She is asymptomatic of a urinary tract infection and is otherwise well.

    What is the most appropriate action?

    A   Antibiotics and send urine for culture
    B   Blood tests including a full blood count and renal function
    C   Renal ultrasound scan and antibiotics
    D   Routine urine dipstick at next appointment
    E   Send urine for culture and treat if positive

3. A 22-year-old primiparous woman books her pregnancy at 11 weeks' gestation. Her booking blood tests reveal a haemoglobin level of 10.1 g/dL. Electrophoresis reveals haemoglobin karyotype HbAS.

    What is the diagnosis?

    A   Beta-thalassaemia major
    B   Beta-thalassaemia trait
    C   Hereditary spherocytosis
    D   Sickle cell anaemia
    E   Sickle cell trait

4. A 32-year-old woman is being continuously monitored during labour using a cardiotocograph (CTG). She has had one previous caesarean section for breech presentation at term. She is at 40 weeks' gestation and in spontaneous labour. The baseline of the CTG is 115 beats per minute.

    Regarding CTG analysis, what is the accepted range for a reassuring/normal baseline rate?

    A   80–100 beats per minute
    B   90–120 beats per minute
    C   110–140 beats per minute
    D   100–160 beats per minute
    E   120–180 beats per minute

5. A 32-year-old multiparous pregnant woman attends the antenatal clinic for review at 28 weeks' gestation. She mentions that her 4-year-old daughter has chickenpox. She is unsure whether she has had chickenpox before.

    Serology results revealed the following:

    Varicella zoster virus IgM: negative

    Varicella zoster virus IgG: positive

    What do the serology results suggest regarding her immune status with respect to chickenpox?

    A   Acute episode of shingles
    B   Varicella zoster – chronic carrier
    C   Varicella zoster – current acute infection
    D   Varicella zoster – no acute infection, no previous exposure
    E   Varicella zoster – previous exposure

6. A 40-year-old primiparous woman is admitted and investigated for raised blood pressure. Urine dipstick reveals protein 3+. A 24-hour urine collection is sent for protein calculation.

    What level of urinary protein excretion in 24-hour indicates significant proteinuria?

    A   > 0.1 g
    B   > 0.2 g
    C   > 0.3 g
    D   > 0.4 g
    E   > 0.5 g

7. A 27-year-old primiparous woman presents with mild abdominal pain and some vaginal spotting. Her last menstrual period was 5 weeks ago. Her serum β-human chorionic gonadotrophin (β-hCG) on presentation is 258 IU/L. As she is clinically stable with no risk factors for ectopic pregnancy, she goes home and returns to the early pregnancy unit 2 days later for a repeat serum β-hCG. Her day 3 serum β-hCG is 460 IU/L.

Which of the statements below best describes this patient's serum β-hCG trend?

A   Normal rise, cannot exclude ectopic pregnancy
B   Normal rise, confirmatory of a viable intrauterine pregnancy
C   Suboptimal rise, suggestive of early miscarriage
D   Suboptimal rise, suggestive of ectopic pregnancy
E   None of the above

8. A couple with primary subfertility, who have been trying to conceive for over 12 months, attend a reproductive medicine clinic. The male partner has already given a semen sample for analysis.

The results of semen analysis are as follows:

Normal morphology: 15%

Volume: 4.5 mL

Sperm count: 8 million sperm/mL

Total motility: 61%

What does this analysis indicate?

A   Normal semen analysis
B   Reduced normal morphology, with all other parameters normal
C   Reduced sperm count, with all other parameters normal
D   Reduced total motility, with all other parameters normal
E   Reduced volume, with all other parameters normal

9. A 34-year-old primiparous woman is induced at 40 weeks' gestation and 12 days for post-dates. The fetus is being continuously monitored via a cardiotocograph (CTG). At 6 cm dilatation the CTG becomes pathological and fetal blood samples (FBS) are taken.

The results of the FBS are as follows:

Sample 1: pH 7.19

Sample 2: pH 7.20

What is the most appropriate interpretation and action based on the FBS results?

A   Abnormal result, consider immediate delivery of baby
B   Abnormal result, repeat sample within 30 minutes if CTG remains pathological
C   Borderline result, repeat within 30 minutes if CTG remains pathological
D   Normal result, no further action required
E   Normal result, repeat sample within 1 hour if CTG remains pathological

10. A 23-year-old woman is admitted at 6 weeks' gestation with severe hyperemesis gravidarum. Her serum potassium is 2.7 mmol/L.

What is the normal range of serum potassium?

A   2.5–3.0 mmol/L

B   2.7–3.5 mmol/L
C   3.0–4.0 mmol/L
D   3.5–5.0 mmol/L
E   4.0–5.5 mmol/L

11. A 64-year-old woman undergoes a total abdominal hysterectomy and bilateral salpingo-oophorectomy for endometrial carcinoma. The staging of the specimen is described as stage Ib.

   What is the definition of stage Ib endometrial cancer?

   A   Endocervical invasion only
   B   Extension to adjacent organs
   C   Extension to vagina
   D   Less than half the myometrial depth invaded
   E   Limited to endometrium

12. An 82-year-old woman is undergoing investigation for postmenopausal bleeding. Her serum lactate dehydrogenase (LDH) is raised.

   Which of the following conditions is associated with a normal level of LDH?

   A   Haemolysis
   B   Myocardial infarction
   C   Paget's disease
   D   Pulmonary embolism
   E   Tumour necrosis

13. A 54-year-old woman is investigated for abdominal bloating and weight loss. Blood tests are sent as part of her investigations.

   Which of the following serum levels would be increased if the she had hepatocellular cancer?

   A   Alpha-fetoprotein
   B   CA15-3
   C   Carcinoembryonic antigen
   D   Creatinine kinase
   E   Neurone specific enolase

14. A 67-year-old woman is undergoing investigation for postmenopausal bleeding. An ultrasound scan shows her endometrial thickness to be 6mm.

   What is considered a normal endometrial thickness for a postmenopausal woman?

   A   <2 mm
   B   <3 mm
   C   <4 mm
   D   <6 mm
   E   <8 mm

15. A 32-year-old primiparous woman attends the maternity day unit at 34 weeks' gestation complaining of itching of the palms of her hands. Her blood tests show raised bile acids of 17 µmol/L. Her alanine aminotransferase is raised to 180 IU/L.

What is the most likely diagnosis?

A   Alcoholic liver disease
B   Dermatitis
C   Gallstones
D   Hepatitis B
E   Obstetric cholestasis

16. A 38-year-old woman attends a colposcopy clinic following an abnormal result of moderate dyskaryosis at cervical screening. The results of the biopsy taken at colposcopy indicate cervical intraepithelial neoplasia (CIN) II.

What is the extent of cervical involvement in CIN II?

A   1/4 thickness of squamous epithelium affected
B   1/3 thickness of squamous epithelium affected
C   2/3 thickness of squamous epithelium affected
D   Full thickness of squamous epithelium affected
E   None of the above

17. A 25-year-old nulliparous woman attends cervical screening for the first time. The results of her smear test show borderline nuclear changes.

What is the appropriate follow-up for this woman?

A   Immediate referral to colposcopy
B   Repeat smear in 1 year
C   Repeat smear in 3 years
D   Repeat smear in 3 months
E   Repeat smear in 6 months

18. A 25-year-old primiparous woman has a forceps delivery. She sustains trauma to the perineum. You perform as per rectal examination. You note that < 50% of the thickness of the external sphincter has been torn.

What grade of perineal tear has the patient sustained?

A   Fourth degree tear
B   Second degree tear
C   Third degree tear – class A
D   Third degree tear – class B
E   Third degree tear – class C

19. A 38-year-old multiparous woman is admitted with a heavy antepartum haemorrhage (APH) at 26 weeks' gestation. She has had three previous caesarean sections. On examination, her abdomen is soft and non-tender.

What is the most likely cause of this woman's APH?

A   Abruption
B   Placenta praevia
C   Trauma
D   Vasa praevia
E   Uterine rupture

20. A 32-year-old primiparous woman with gestational diabetes is 32 weeks pregnant. At her antenatal clinic review, her symphysis fundal height is measured as 38 cm. She is referred for an urgent scan to assess fetal growth and amniotic fluid index.

Which amniotic fluid index would indicate polyhydramnios?

A ≥ 5 cm
B ≥ 10 cm
C ≥ 15 cm
D ≥ 18 cm
E ≥ 22 cm

Answers

1. A A repeat sample should be performed in 30 minutes

This fetal blood sample (FBS) shows a pH of 7.24, which is classified as suspicious. The sample should be repeated in no more than 30 minutes, or sooner if clinically indicated. See **Table 10.1** for a FBS action plan.

Table 10.1 Interpretation of fetal blood sampling (FBS) results		
Result (pH)	**Interpretation**	**Action**
≥ 7.25	Normal	Repeat FBS if cardiotocograph remains pathological or suspicious
7.21–7.24	Suspicious	Repeat FBS in 30 minutes or sooner if indicated
≤ 7.20	Abnormal	Delivery

2. E Send urine for culture and treat if positive

Urine tract infection (UTI) is defined as the presence of 100,000/mL organisms in an asymptomatic patient or 100/mL organisms with increased white cell count in a symptomatic patient. In an asymptomatic patient, the diagnosis of a urinary tract infection should be made once the presence of a pathogen has been confirmed on culture. Asymptomatic bacteriuria is the presence of 100,000/mL of organisms in the absence of symptoms on at least two occasions. These are treated as there is a risk of cystitis and ascending infection which may increase maternal or fetal morbidity.

Urinalysis should be performed on pregnant women routinely at all antenatal clinic visits. The presence of protein, leucocytes and nitrites can suggest the presence of a UTI. A renal ultrasound scan would only be indicated in the presence of recurrent pyelonephritis or if renal abnormality or disease is suspected.

3. E Sickle cell trait

Sickle cell conditions are due to the production of abnormal β peptide chains leading to abnormal haemoglobin. The gene which codes for the β chain of haemoglobin has an amino acid substitution which results in the production of HbS rather than HbA. Individuals with sickle cell anaemia are homozygous with HbSS. Heterozygotes have HbAS and have sickle cell trait. Sickle cell trait is thought to be protective against *Plasmodium falciparum* malaria. Sickle cell anaemia results in the production of fragile erythrocytes which leads to their early destruction and subsequent haemolysis. In sickle cell trait there may be mild anaemia, but there is usually no evidence of haemolysis, i.e. normal lactate dehydrogenase, bilirubin and a normal reticulocyte count. Ideally these patients should have pre-pregnancy counselling and screening of their partner. If this has not been undertaken prior to conception, then it should be arranged as soon as it is identified to determine the risk of HbSS in the fetus.

4. D 100–160 beats per minute

Cardiotocography (CTG) or electronic fetal monitoring is commonly used during pregnancy and labour to determine fetal well-being. A range of parameters are studied including baseline fetal heart rate which is considered normal if between 100–160 beats per minute. Fetal cardiac activity is controlled via the sympathetic and parasympathetic autonomic nervous systems, with other influences coming from oxygenation and baroreceptors. Fetal baseline heart rate generally falls as the pregnancy increases and this is a result of the parasympathetic system becoming more developed. Developing intrapartum fetal tachycardia, when associated with maternal tachycardia, may be as a result of infection and chorioamnionitis should be considered.

National Institute for Health and Clinical Excellence. Intrapartum Care for Healthy Women and Babies. Clinical Guidance CG190. London: NICE, 2014.

5. E Varicella zoster – previous exposure

Varicella zoster virus is a member of the herpes virus family and causes chickenpox. The majority of adults in the UK are immune to chickenpox. It is transmitted via droplet infection and has a relatively long incubation period of approximately 2 weeks. Chickenpox infection is more severe in pregnancy and there is a higher rate of complications, such as varicella pneumonitis. Once there has been exposure to the virus there will be initial production of varicella IgM antibodies, followed by the production of long-term immunity through IgG antibodies. In the case illustrated, the patient has IgG positive result and is therefore immune to varicella zoster through previous exposure. There is therefore no risk to the fetus and no indication for immunoglobulin. If IgM was positive and IgG negative, this would suggest recent infection with no prior immunity and this would be an indication for immunoglobulin.

6. C >0.3 g

Urinary protein excretion of >0.3 g in 24 hours indicates a significant level of proteinuria. This may be found in conditions such as pre-eclampsia or pre-existing renal disease. Severe proteinuria may not always be associated with significantly raised blood pressure and may be due to long-standing renal damage and should be investigated.

7. A Normal rise, cannot exclude ectopic pregnancy

When serum β-human chorionic gonadotrophin (β-hCG) is 1500 IU/L it is unlikely that an intrauterine pregnancy will be seen on transvaginal ultrasound scan. Serum β-hCG monitoring is used to aid the management and diagnosis of women in early pregnancy with symptoms of suggestive of early miscarriage or ectopic pregnancy when scanning is unlikely to yield little useful information. A normal rise in serum β-hCG is that of at least 66% every 48 hours. Although a normal rise over 48 hours is suggestive of a normal pregnancy it remains a pregnancy of unknown location until there has been a confirmatory scan. A β-hCG that is falling may indicate both a failing intrauterine or failing ectopic pregnancy. A suboptimal rise in β-hCG, i.e. a rise that is < 66% over 48 hours, increases suspicion of an ectopic pregnancy; however, it does not rule out the presence of an intrauterine pregnancy.

8. C Reduced sperm count, with all other parameters normal

The World Health Organization (WHO) has defined the normal reference ranges for semen analysis. A minimum of 15 million sperm/mL is acceptable as per the WHO. This man's sperm count is only 8 million sperm/mL and is therefore considered to be suboptimal. A minimum of 4% of semen with normal morphology is acceptable. The lowest acceptable volume of the ejaculate is 1.5 mL. The total motility of a sample refers to the percentage of both progressive and non-progressive forms. The WHO considers 40% to be the minimum acceptable percentage for total motility. For the most accurate results analysis should be performed within 60 minutes of production.

Cooper TG, Noonan E, von Eckardstein S, et al. World Health Organization reference values for human semen characteristics. Hum Reprod Update 2010; 16:231–245.

9. A Abnormal result, consider immediate delivery of baby

Fetal blood sampling (FBS) is a means of assessing fetal well-being when there are concerns raised when using electronic fetal monitoring during labour. The results of fetal blood samples are used to assess fetal hypoxia in the presence of an accompanying pathological cardiotocograph (CTG). The normal fetal blood pH range is 7.25–7.35. If a sample is within this range in the presence of a pathological CTG then a further FBS sample should be taken within 1 hour if the CTG remains pathological. When the pH obtained is between 7.21 and 7.24 the result is classified as borderline and a repeat sample should be taken within 30 minutes if the CTG remains pathological. A sample with a pH of 7.20 or less is considered abnormal and therefore immediate delivery of the baby should be considered.

10. D 3.5–5.0 mmol/L

The normal range for potassium in an adult human is 3.5–5.0 mmol/L. This value may vary between hospitals. Hypokalaemia is a common abnormality in hyperemesis gravidarum as a result of persistent vomiting and should be corrected to avoid complications of hypokalaemia.

11. D Less than half the myometrial depth invaded

Endometrial cancer is classified according to the extent of tumour invasion.

Stage I: limited to uterus

- a: limited to endometrium

- b: less half myometrial depth
- c: greater than half myometrial depth

Stage II: tumour in uterine body and cervix

Stage III: extended to uterine serosa, peritoneal cavity +/– lymph nodes

Stage IV: extended outside the pelvis, may involve bladder or bowel

12. C Paget's disease

Lactate dehydrogenase is a plasma enzyme that may be raised in the following conditions:

- Active liver disease
- Haemolysis
- Pulmonary embolism
- Myocardial infarction

It is not associated with Paget's disease; alkaline phosphatase is raised in Paget's disease.

13. A Alpha-fetoprotein

Alpha-fetoprotein is increased in hepatocellular cancer and active liver disease. CA 15-3 is a non-specific tumour marker which may be raised in breast cancer. Carcinoembryonic is generally increased in abdominal and gastric cancers. It may also be increased in cirrhosis. Neurone-specific enolase is raised in small cell cancer of the lungs.

14. C <4 mm

Bleeding after the menopause is a common presentation and should initially be investigated using transvaginal ultrasound scan. An endometrial thickness of ≥ 4 mm is abnormal and should be followed up with endometrial sampling, which may be via pipelle biopsy or hysteroscopy. The majority of women with postmenopausal bleeding are found to have atrophic endometrium. Polyps, hyperplasia or malignant change may also be found.

15. E Obstetric cholestasis

Obstetric cholestasis is a condition that is unique to pregnancy. It is characterised by pruritus, abnormal liver enzymes and raised bile acids. It should be considered a diagnosis of exclusion. There is thought to be a genetic link and a predisposition to the cholestatic effect of increased circulating oestrogen. Treatment is to control the symptoms with antihistamines and ursodeoxycholic acid. There should be increased fetal surveillance and consideration of delivery from 37 weeks' gestation as there is an association with intrauterine fetal death after 37/40 weeks.

16. C 2/3 thickness of squamous epithelium affected

Cervical intraepithelial neoplasia (CIN) is the term given to describe the histological changes associated with dysplasia that may occur in the cervix. CIN is considered the precursor of cervical cancer. The grading of CIN is based on the thickness of the squamous epithelium affected (from the basal layer of the transformation zone upwards). CIN I is the mildest form, only affecting the bottom third of the basal layer, CIN II affects the bottom two-thirds of the squamous epithelium, whereas CIN III is the most severe form of CIN and refers to changes affecting more than two-thirds to full thickness of the epithelium (**Table 10.2**).

Table 10.2 Cervical intraepithelial neoplasia (CIN) categories and histology	
Grade	**Thickness of squamous epithelium affected**
CIN I	Basal 1/3
CIN II	Bottom 2/3
CIN III	> 2/3 to full thickness

17. E Repeat smear in 6 months

Borderline nuclear changes on cervical screening are suggestive of cervical intraepithelial neoplasia (CIN) II to III affecting some of the cells sampled. It is appropriate for this woman to have a repeat smear test in 6 months' time. If she was to have a total of three consecutive smears with the same result she would need to be referred with colposcopy. A similar recall of 6 months would also be appropriate for a result showing inflammatory changes on smear. The standard recall for a normal smear test result is 3 years. More severe changes smear, i.e. mild, moderate or severe dyskaryosis indicate the need for colposcopy.

18. C Third degree tear – class A

This woman has sustained a third degree perineal tear. This means that the tear is severe enough as to involve the anal sphincter. Third degree tears can be graded A–C, according to the extent of trauma to the external and internal anal sphincters. In a third degree A (3a) tear < 50% of the thickness of the external anal sphincter has been damaged. A third degree B (3b) tear describes a tear damaging more than 50% of the thickness of the external anal sphincter. When the internal anal sphincter has been damaged (to any extent) the tear is classified as a third degree C (3c) tear. A fourth degree tear involves damage to the anal epithelium, in addition to any third degree tear. A first-degree tear is considered to be a minor injury to the perineal skin or vaginal epithelium. This superficial injury typically does not require any repair. A second degree tear is one where the vaginal/perineal muscles are torn, whilst maintaining the integrity of the anal sphincter.

19. B Placenta praevia

Placenta praevia is a common cause of antepartum haemorrhage. It is classified as either minor placenta praevia or major placenta praevia. Minor placenta praevia is as placenta which has inserted into the lower segment of the uterus, but does not cover the cervical os. Major placenta praevia (previously classified as grade III and grade IV) describes placental position when the placenta covers the cervical os. Risk factors for placenta praevia include previous caesarean section, multiple pregnancy and maternal age. The majority of antepartum haemorrhages are idiopathic. Other causes include placental abruption, vasa praevia and local cervical or vaginal pathologies.

20. E ≥ 22 cm

Polyhydramnios is an overall increase in liquor volume. It may be diagnosed if the deepest pool of fluid seen on ultrasound scan is deeper than 8 cm or if the overall amniotic fluid index (AFI) is > 22 cm. Causes of polyhydramnios include diabetes and fetal anomalies causing problems with swallowing and idiopathic causes.

Chapter 11

Immunology

Questions

For each question, select the single best answer from the five options listed.

1. A female baby is born via spontaneous vaginal delivery at term. As she is born in an urban area with high levels of tuberculosis she is given the BCG (Bacillus Calmette–Guerin) vaccination before she is taken home by her parents.

    What type of vaccine is the BCG vaccine?

    A Conjugate vaccine
    B Killed (inactivated) vaccine
    C Live (attenuated) vaccine
    D Subunit vaccine
    E Toxoid vaccine

2. Which of the following is an example of a disease caused by type III hypersensitivity?

    A Asthma
    B Autoimmune haemolytic anaemia
    C Eczema
    D Multiple sclerosis
    E Systemic lupus erythematosus

3. Which of the following is most important in the adaptive immune system?

    A Complement
    B Macrophages
    C Natural killer cells
    D Neutrophils
    E T-helper cells

4. One of the known benefits of breastfeeding is its role in supporting the infant's immune system.

    Which of the following antibodies is secreted in large amounts in breast milk?

    A IgA
    B IgD
    C IgE
    D IgG
    E IgM

5. At her booking appointment a pregnant woman is found to be rubella non-immune.

    What type of vaccine is rubella?

    A   Conjugated
    B   Live attenuated
    C   Inactivated
    D   Subunit
    E   Toxoid

6. A patient who is allergic to penicillin is erroneously given a penicillin-containing antibiotic and develops an acute allergic reaction.

    What type of hypersensitivity reaction is this?

    A   Type 1
    B   Type 2
    C   Type 3
    D   Type 4
    E   Type 5

7. The human leucocyte antigen (HLA) system is responsible for regulation of the immune system.

    At which gene is the HLA system based?

    A   Chromosome 2
    B   Chromosome 5
    C   Chromosome 6
    D   Chromosome 10
    E   Chromosome 11

8. Which type of cells are the most effective at antigen presenting in immune response?

    A   Dendritic cells
    B   Monocytes
    C   Macrophages
    D   Interleukin
    E   Natural killer cells

Answers

---

1. C Live (attenuated) vaccine

Attenuated vaccines contain live but attenuated organisms. That is, they lack the ability to be pathogenic, but will initiate an immune response. Examples of live (attenuated) vaccines are MMR (mumps, measles, rubella), polio (Sabin) and Bacillus Calmette–Guérin. Killed (inactivated) vaccines are generally considered more stable and safer than live vaccines. However, as the immune response to killed vaccines is generally weaker than to live vaccines, adjuvants such as aluminium hydroxide are added to the killed vaccine in order to precipitate an improved immune response. Examples of killed (inactivated) vaccines include the hepatitis A, pertussis, influenza and polio (Salk) vaccines. Toxoid vaccines confer immunity by the administration of inactivated toxin. Examples include the tetanus and diphtheria vaccines, which are often given in combination. Subunit vaccines use specific antigens, in order to elicit an appropriate immune response. The hepatitis B vaccine is one such subunit vaccine.

---

2. E Systemic lupus erythematosus

Type III hypersensitivity is also known as immune complex hypersensitivity. It refers to a failure of immune complex clearance, leading to their deposition in tissues. In this form of hypersensitivity, there is a failure to clear antibody-antigen complexes (usually IgG). These complexes initiate the complement cascade, activate neutrophils and macrophages and lead to platelet aggregation. This inflammatory reaction may lead to a vasculitis in the surrounding tissues. The complex deposition may have a systemic effect or be localised to an organ. Systemic lupus erythematosus is an example of a condition in which there is multiple organ immune complex deposition leading to manifestations such as arthritis, rashes, lupus nephritis and myocarditis. Type III hypersensitivity is also responsible for conditions such as serum sickness, post-streptococcal glomerulonephritis, rheumatoid arthritis, extrinsic allergic alveolitis and the Arthus reaction, whereby immune complex deposition results in localised vasculitis at the site of an injection, e.g. after a tetanus vaccination.

---

3. E T-helper cells

The innate immune system provides immediate and non-specific response to attack, whereas the adaptive immune system provides a more complex and specific response to antigens and generates immunological memory. Central to the rapid response (within hours) of the innate immune system is the complement cascade.

Complement proteins are mainly made by the liver and provide a type of immune defence; marking antigens for destruction by other cells (through opsonisation), recruiting other elements of the innate immune system, such as macrophages and neutrophils, assisting antibodies (part of the acquired immune system) and also by aiding the removal of immune complexes. Natural killer cells are part of the innate immune system and provide a non-specific response. This response is particularly strong against tumour cells and viruses due to their cytotoxic activity. Programmed cell death takes place in target cells as a result of the release of cytotoxic granules, such as perforin. T-helper cells are a specialised type of lymphocytes and therefore part of the adaptive or acquired immune system; in particular they play an important role in activating B-lymphocytes.

4. A IgA

Antibodies, or immunoglobulins, are glycoproteins produced by B cells as part of the acquired immune system. The 'default' form of antibody is IgM, however each form of antibody has a specialised function, and are therefore differentially distributed in line with their role in immunity (**Table 11.1**). The key to the acquired immune system is the ability of B cells to switch class of antibody production in response to the attacking antigen. IgA has key role in mucosal immunity and is therefore the predominant antibody present in bodily secretions such as saliva, colostrum, tears and is found in high concentrations in the respiratory, reproductive and gastrointestinal tracts. Key to its functionality in inferring immunity to the neonate is IgA's resistance to stomach acid; this enables the capacity for IgA to be secreted in breast milk and benefit the infant from its mother's immunological memory.

Table 11.1 Antibodies and their properties

Antibody	Properties	Additional properties
IgA	Protects mucosal surfaces	Secreted in breast milk, tears, saliva, etc.
IgD	Role uncertain	Found in serum
IgE	Activates mast cells	Involved in allergic response and anaphylaxis
IgG	Fixes complement Opsonising properties	Crosses placenta
IgM	Fixes complement Opsonising properties	Default antibody, i.e. first made

5. B Live attenuated

It is recommended that before pregnancy, women are up to date with all of the routine adult vaccines, in particular measles, mumps and rubella (MMR).

This is a table summarising different vaccination types and their suitability in pregnancy:

Live attenuated vaccines	MMR Varicella Influenza (nasal)	Avoid during pregnancy and one month before conception. Can give immediately postpartum, if indicated.
Inactivated/Toxoid	Influenza (vaccine) Tetanus, diphtheria and acelluar pertussis booster vaccine (Tdap) Hepatitis A Human papillomavirus (HPV) Hepatitis B Meningococcal	Can be given before or after pregnancy, if indicated.

Pregnant women are advised to have the whooping cough vaccination (Tdap booster) in every pregnancy, ideally between 27–36th weeks. This will provide the greatest protection to the newborn baby in early life before they receive their first whooping cough vaccine (DTaP) at 2 months old. It is estimated that 30–40% of babies who get whooping cough catch it from their mother, when a source is identified.

6. A Type 1

There are four types of hypersensitivity reactions:

Type 1 reactions, also known as immediate hypersensitivity reactions, include anaphylaxis, atopy and allergic asthma. They are caused by IgE-mediated degranulation of mast cells, triggered by antigen binding. Clinical signs are apparent in less than 30 minutes.

Type 2 reactions are cytotoxic and include transfusion reactions and rhesus incompatibility. Antigens cause formation of IgM and IgG antibodies that bind to the surface of the target cell and are then destroyed by complement. Clinical signs appear within 5–12 hours.

Type 3 reactions are immune complex mediated. Antibody-antigen complexes are deposited in tissues leading to local or systemic inflammation. Diseases include rheumatoid arthritis and systemic lupus erythematosus (SLE). Clinical signs appear within 3–8 hours.

Type 4 reactions are delayed types of hypersensitivity. Activated type-1 T-helper cells release cytokines, leading to macrophage and cytotoxic T cell accumulation. Examples include contact dermatitis and chronic transplant rejection. Clinical signs are apparent within 24–48 hours.

7. C Chromosome 6

The human leucocyte antigen (HLA) is a set of genes found on chromosome 6. The HLA bind to fragments from pathogens and display them on the cell surface for T-cell recognition, thus regulating the immune system. Different HLAs correspond to the three classes of major histocompatibility complex (MHC). MHC class 1 are displayed on cells, which are containing foreign proteins and are recognised by cytotoxic (CD-8) T-cells. Class 2 are expressed on B-cells and recognised by helper (CD-4) T-cells. Class 3 are involved in the regulation of the complement cascade.

8. A Dendritic Cells

Dendritic cells originate from the bone marrow and are the most efficient antigen-presenting cell (APC). They acquire antigens in the blood stream and tissues and process them in the lymphoid organs, which triggers an immunological response.

Macrophages may also function as APCs by ingesting foreign material and presenting it to T and B-cells.

Monocytes are produced by the bone marrow and circulate in the bloodstream for one to three days before migrating into tissues where they differentiate into dendritic cells or macrophages.

Interleukins are a group of cytokines produced in response to inflammation and infection. They promote development and differentiation of T and B-lymphocytes.

Natural killer cells are effector cells, which can directly kill virus-infected cells and certain tumours.

Chapter 12

Microbiology

Questions

For each question, select the single best answer from the five options listed.

1. Antenatal screening of a 25-year-old patient is suggestive of hepatitis B infection. The results of her serology are as follows:

HBsAg	Positive
HBeAg	Positive
Anti-HBeAb	Negative
Anti-HBsAb	Negative
Total anti-HBc	Positive (IgM anti-core Ab negative, IgG anti-core Ab positive)

    Which of the following is most likely to represent her hepatitis B status?

    A   Acute infection (recent)
    B   Acute infection (resolving)
    C   Chronic infection (high infectivity)
    D   Chronic infection (low infectivity)
    E   Following vaccination

2. A 23-year-old woman attends antenatal clinic at 22 weeks' gestation. This is her second pregnancy and she is very concerned as during her first pregnancy she had an 'infection', which led to the permanent disability of her child. He is deaf, with delayed development and is small for his age. He became jaundiced shortly after birth.

    What was the most likely cause of her son's condition?

    A   Cytomegalovirus
    B   Herpes
    C   Parvovirus B19
    D   Rubella
    E   Varicella zoster

3. A 38-year-old woman from Sri Lanka attends her general practitioner at 10 weeks' gestation. She is complaining of fever and has pains in her joints. She developed a rash yesterday. On examination, she has a temperature of 38.1°C, postauricular lymphadenopathy and a maculopapular rash over her torso. Rubella is diagnosed.

What is the most likely fetal abnormality to occur as a result of this acute infection?

A   Cerebral palsy
B   Failure to thrive
C   Limb hypoplasia
D   Microcephaly
E   Sensorineural hearing loss

4.   A 15-year-old girl attends the genitourinary medicine clinic complaining of vaginal itching and green vaginal discharge. She is sexually active with her 17-year-old boyfriend and uses the oral contraceptive pill. Speculum examination reveals haemorrhages on her cervix. A urine pregnancy test is negative.

Considering the most likely diagnosis, what is the most appropriate first line antibiotic?

A   Azithromycin 1 g once only
B   Doxycycline 100 mg twice daily + metronidazole 400 mg three times daily + ofloxacin 400 mg twice daily for 7 days
C   Doxycycline 100 mg twice daily for 14 days + metronidazole 400 mg three times daily for 7 days
D   Metronidazole 400 mg three times daily for 5 days
E   Tinidazole 2 g once only

5.   Which of the following is an obligate anaerobic organism?

A   *Bacteroides*
B   *Escherichia coli*
C   *Listeria*
D   *Mycobacteria*
E   *Pseudomonas*

6.   A 23-year-old woman attends her general practitioner complaining of numbness and tingling in both feet. She recently started treatment for pulmonary tuberculosis.

Which drug is most likely to be responsible for these symptoms?

A   Ethambutol
B   Isoniazid
C   Pyrazinamide
D   Rifampicin
E   Streptomycin

7.   A 38-year-old woman is readmitted via the emergency department 10 days post emergency caesarean section complaining of vaginal bleeding, abdominal pain and foul-smelling vaginal discharge. Abdominal examination reveals suprapubic tenderness and the uterus is palpable 2 cm below the umbilicus. You suspect endometritis.

Which of the following is the most likely causative organism?

A   *Chlamydia trachomatis*
B   Group B *Streptococcus*
C   *Mycoplasma genitalia*
D   *Neisseria gonorrhoea*
E   *Ureaplasma*

8. A woman presents at 28 weeks' gestation with vomiting, headache, night sweats and abdominal pain. She has recently returned from the African country of Mali. Urgent blood films show the presence of *Plasmodium falciparum*, with a parasitaemia of 3%. After a diagnosis of malaria has been made she is treated with intravenous quinine.

The presence of which haematological characteristic is associated with increased incidence of malaria?

A   Haemoglobin C
B   Beta-thalassaemia
C   Duffy antigen
D   Glucose-6-phosphate dehydrogenase deficiency
E   Sickle cell trait

9. What is Group B β-haemolytic *Streptococcus* also known as?

A   *Streptococcus agalactiae*
B   *Streptococcus anginosus*
C   *Streptococcus pneumoniae*
D   *Streptococcus pyogenes*
E   *Streptococcus viridans*

10. A 34-year-old nulliparous woman presents at 39 weeks' gestation in labour, following spontaneous rupture of membranes. It is noted that a high vaginal swab taken during the pregnancy was positive for Group B β-haemolytic *Streptococcus*. She is clinically well and there are no signs of fetal distress.

What is the appropriate antimicrobial regimen to give this patient?

A   Intravenous ampicillin 500 mg QDS
B   Intravenous co-amoxiclav 1.5 g TDS
C   Intravenous benzylpenicillin 3 g, then 1.5 g every 4 hours
D   Intravenous piperacillin/tazobactam 4.5 g TDS
E   Oral erythromycin 250 mg QDS

11. Which of the following bacteria produces an endotoxin?

A   *Clostridium botulinum*
B   *Clostridium tetani*
C   *Escheridia coli*
D   *Neisseria meningitidis*
E   *Staphylococcus aureus*

12. Which of the following is a DNA virus?

    A Hepatitis A
    B Hepatitis B
    C Hepatitis C
    D Hepatitis D
    E Hepatitis E

13. Which of the following is a Gram-positive genus of bacterium?

    A *Clostridium*
    B *Haemophilus*
    C *Legionella*
    D *Salmonella*
    E *Shigella*

14. Which of the following is the causative agent of Cytomegalovirus in humans?

    A Human herpesvirus 1
    B Human herpesvirus 5
    C Human herpesvirus 6
    D Human herpesvirus 7
    E Human herpesvirus 8

Answers

1. C Chronic infection (high infectivity)

Hepatitis B is a double-stranded DNA virus. The virus is responsible for causing jaundice, hepatitis, cirrhosis and an increased risk of hepatocellular carcinoma. The virus may be spread via sexual intercourse, exposure to infected blood (i.e. shared needles) or vertically from mother to child. The presence of HBs-antigen (HBsAg) indicates infection; HBsAg is typically present for the first 6 months after infection; however, if it persists beyond this then infection is considered chronic. The presence of HBeAg shows viral replication and therefore high infectivity. Anti-HBc is produced soon after infection (initially as IgM, then as IgG) and indicates previous or ongoing infection. Anti-HBsAb indicates previous exposure and is positive after vaccination and in cases where infection has been cleared by the immune system with subsequent immunity. In this patient there is evidence of chronic infection with ongoing high infectivity. The baby will likely need immunising against hepatitis B and specific immunoglobulin at birth and the neonatologist should be informed.

2. A Cytomegalovirus

Cytomegalovirus (CMV) is the most common congenital infection. Pregnant women often do not realise they have the infection as it is frequently asymptomatic. Approximately 5–10% of congenitally infected babies have symptoms apparent at birth which, if present, is a poor prognostic sign. Ten per cent of babies affected at birth die and one-third develop cerebral palsy. Of the babies who are not symptomatic at birth, approximately 1 in 6 are deaf, 1 in 10 have developmental delay and 1% suffer from retinitis.

3. E Sensorineural hearing loss

Rubella causes most problems if it is contracted during the first trimester, leading to miscarriage in up to 20% of cases. If miscarriage does not occur, there is a strong possibility that the fetus will be affected in some way. Approximately, 70% will suffer sensorineural hearing loss, 50% suffer retinopathy and eye abnormalities and 40% may suffer from congenital heart abnormalities, such as a patent ductus arteriosus and ventricular septal defects. This woman should have her serology sent urgently.

The virus is excreted in pharyngeal secretions during the incubation period for up to 7 days before the appearance of the rash.

4. D Metronidazole 400 mg three times daily for 5 days

Trichomonas vaginalis is a sexually transmitted infection of the lower genital tract caused by a protozoa. Symptoms include itching and inflammation of the vulva and vagina. There is often purulent vaginal discharge and the cervix may have the classic haemorrhages giving it the classic description of a 'strawberry cervix'.

Swabs should be sent for culture and other sexually transmitted diseases should always be considered. Trichomonas is a rare cause of pelvic inflammatory disease, however contact tracing is necessary. First line treatment is metronidazole, either 2 g as a single dose or 400 mg three times a day for 5 days. Sexual intercourse should be avoided until treatment is completed in the patient and also the partner, if necessary. This patient should be advised that while the oral contraceptive pill is effective for preventing pregnancy, barrier methods should also be used to prevent sexually transmitted infections. Treatment with metronidazole would be safe in pregnancy.

5. A *Bacteroides*

Obligate anaerobes are organisms that live and thrive in the absence of oxygen; they will die in the presence of oxygen. Examples include *Bacteroides*, *Clostridium* and *Actinomyces*. By contrast, a facultative anaerobe is able to alter its function depending on the presence or absence of oxygen. Examples include *Staphylococcus aureus*, *Escherichia coli* and *Listeria*.

6. B Isoniazid

Tuberculosis (TB) has a prevalence in the UK of 15–50/100,000 population, depending on the location. The highest levels are currently in London. The disease most commonly affects the lungs and 60% of infected individuals having pulmonary involvement. TB may affect other organs including the genitourinary tract, which may present with a pelvic mass or chronic pelvic inflammatory disease. This occurs as a result of haematogenous spread from the primary location. Treatment of TB involves 6 months of medication with rifampicin, isoniazid and pyrazinamide. Ethambutol has recently been added to address the issue of resistance. Side effects of the medication include:

- Rifampicin: orange urine and tears, hepatotoxicity
- Isoniazid: hepatotoxicity, peripheral neuropathy (may be reduced by administration of pyridoxine)
- Pyrazinamide: hepatotoxicity, gout
- Ethambutol: optic neuritis

7. E *Ureaplasma*

Endometritis may be acute or chronic. In this case, the patient has an acute endometritis after caesarean section. Causes to be considered include retained products of conception and ascending infection from the lower genital tract, with prolonged rupture of membranes being a particular risk factor. Acute endometritis from an obstetric cause is most often polymicrobial, involving vaginal commensals. These bacteria include *Ureaplasma*, *Gardnerella* and group B *Streptococcus*. Other bacteria implicated in endometritis are those associated with sexually transmitted infections including chlamydia and gonorrhoea. Treatment includes initial resuscitation and swift administration of broad spectrum antibiotics. Other investigations include a full blood count, C-reactive protein, clotting profile and pelvic ultrasound.

8. C Duffy antigen

Beta-thalassaemia, like many other haemoglobinopathies, is known to confer an element of protection against malaria. The presence of the sickle cell trait is known to reduce the severity of malarial disease, with fewer hospital admissions and reduced parasite densities. This is due to the suboptimal conditions for the parasites caused by low oxygen concentrations in the serum of individuals with the trait. Individuals with haemoglobin C are also less likely to experience severe malaria, due to reduced ability of the parasite to reproduce. The absence of the Duffy factor provides immunity against *Plasmodium vivax*, as it is the Duffy antigen that parasites bind to.

An individual with glucose-6-phosphate dehydrogenase deficiency typically has an enhanced protection against malaria, in particular *Plasmodium falciparum*.

9. A *Streptococcus agalactiae*

Streptococcus agalactiae is more commonly known as Group B β-haemolytic *Streptococcus* (GBS). It is a common commensal in the gastrointestinal tract and is also part of normal vaginal flora in around a third of women. Although maternal vaginal carriage is not harmful in itself there is the risk of transmission to the baby with the potential to cause neonatal sepsis once membranes rupture. GBS may also be associated with chorioamnionitis in the mother.

Streptococci species are Gram-positive bacteria that are classified according to whether they are alpha-haemolytic or beta-haemolytic. Beta-haemolytic species are further classified as belonging to Lancefield groups A to V. *Streptococcus viridans* and *Streptococcus pneumonia* are both alpha-haemolytic species. *Streptococcus pyogenes* is beta-haemolytic species also known as Group A *Streptococcus*. *Streptococcus anginosus* is also known as Group F *Streptococcus*.

10. C Intravenous benzylpenicillin 3 g, then 1.5 g every 4 hours

Vaginal carriage of Group B *Streptococcus* (GBS) is common. This commensal bacteria is present in the vagina and digestive tract of around 28% of women. It is known that carriage during pregnancy may be associated with chorioamnionitis and infection of the neonate.

If GBS has been detected during the current pregnancy, standard practice in the UK is the administration of intrapartum intravenous antibiotic therapy (a typical regimen being 3 g IV Penicillin G, followed by 1.5 g every 4 hours in labour). Broad spectrum antibiotics, such as ampicillin and co-amoxiclav not advised as they may increase the risk of Gram-negative neonatal sepsis.

11. D *Neisseria meningitides*

Endotoxins are lipopolysaccharides produced by Gram-negative bacteria. They are found in the outer membrane of the bacteria along with a substance called lipid

A which, when released during lysis of the bacteria, is responsible for the toxicity. *Neisseria meningitides* is the only Gram-negative bacteria listed. The other bacteria are all Gram-positive bacteria, known to produce exotoxins. **Table 12.1** gives further details.

Table 12.1 Exotoxins and endotoxins		
	Exotoxin	**Endotoxin**
Producing bacteria	Gram-positive Gram-negative	Gram-negative
Release	Extracellular, released	Structural molecule of Gram-negative bacterial cell wall, released on cell death
Examples of action	Tetanus toxins Cholera symptoms *E. coli* *Shigella*	Lipopolysaccharide Lipid A
Antigenicity	Susceptible to antibodies Destroyed by heating	Limited effect of antibodies

12. B Hepatitis B

Viruses contain either deoxyribonucleic acid (DNA) or ribonucleic acid (RNA) as their genetic material, which may be either single-stranded (ss) or double-stranded (ds) (**Table 12.2**). Further classification of their genetic material is dependent on the 'sense' of the strands i.e. whether positive-sense or negative-sense. Hepatitis B is a double-stranded DNA virus, whilst the other hepatitis viruses listed are RNA single-sense viruses.

Table 12.2 Classification of DNA and RNA viruses	
RNA viruses (ss or ds)	**DNA viruses (ss or ds)**
Hepatitis A, C, D, E (ss)	Herpes simplex 1 and 2 (ds)
HIV (ss)	Varicella zoster (ds)
Human T-lymphotrophic virus (ss)	Cytomegalovirus (ds)
Rubella (ss)	Hepatitis B (ds)
Japanese B Virus (ss)	Human papillovirus (ds)
Respiratory syncytial virus (ss)	Epstein–Barr (ds)
Rotavirus (ds)	Parvovirus B19 (ss)
ss = single-stranded, ds = double-stranded	

13. A *Clostridium*

The ability to Gram-stain bacterium allows classification into two major groups, Gram-positive and Gram-negative. A bacterium which has peptidoglycan in its cell wall will take up Gram stain and therefore is considered Gram-positive. In addition to Gram-staining further simple classification of bacterium is based on appearance, whether as cocci (i.e. spherical shaped), bacilli (i.e. rod shaped) and a further classification of coccibacillus (intermediate shape). See **Table 12.3** for further classification detail.

Table 12.3 Classification of bacteria

	Bacilli	Cocci
Gram-positive	*Listeria* species e.g. • *L. monocytogenes* *Clostridium* species, e.g. • *C. botulinum* • *C. difficile* Actinomyces species, e.g. • *A. israelii* *Mycobacterium* species, e.g. • *M. tuberculosis*	*Staphylococcus* species, e.g. • *S. aureus* *Streptococcus* species, e.g. • *S. pneumoniae* • *S. pyogenes* *Enterococcus* species, e.g. • *E. faecalis*
Gram-negative	*Escherichia* species, e.g. • *E. coli* *Enterobacter* species e.g. • *Proteus mirabilis* *Klebsiella* species, e.g. • *K. pneumoniae* *Salmonella* species, e.g. • *S. enterica* *Shigella* species, e.g. • *S. dysenteriae* *Campylobacter* species, e.g. • *C. jejuni* *Legionella* species, e.g. • *L. pneumophila*	*Neisseria* species, e.g. • *N. gonorrhoeae* • *N. meningitidis* **Coccobacilli:** *Bordetella* species, e.g. • *B. pertussis* *Brucella* species *Haemophilus* species, e.g. • *H. influenzae*

14. B Human herpesvirus 5

Cytomegalovirus (CMV) in humans is caused by human herpesvirus 5 and is the most common cause of congenital infection. Previous infection does not offer immunity, as both primary and recurrent infection during pregnancy may lead to congenital infection. The virus is spread through contact with infected body fluids. Both primary and recurrent infection are often asymptomatic. Any symptoms that are experienced are usually vague and include lethargy and fever. There is no CMV vaccine and antiviral drugs are not currently licensed for use to treat CMV infection during pregnancy. Ganciclovir is sometimes used to treat infection in babies and toddlers to help prevent hearing loss associated with contracting CMV at this age.

Human herpesvirus 1 is the causative agent of the common cold-sore. Both human herpesvirus 6 and human herpesvirus 7 are associated with the childhood disease exanthum subitum. Human herpesvirus 8 is associated with Karposi's sarcoma, which typically occurs in patients with AIDS.

Chapter 13

Pathology

Questions

For each question, select the single best answer from the five options listed.

1. A 27-year-old nulliparous woman and her husband have a series of routine investigations to investigate primary subfertility. She has a hysterosalpingogram which shows she has a bicornuate uterus.

   Which obstetric phenomenon is of increased prevalence in women with a bicornuate uterus?

   A Breech presentation
   B Stillbirth
   C Postpartum haemorrhage
   D Placenta praevia
   E Placenta accrete

2. A 31-year-old nulliparous woman has heavy bleeding at 8 weeks' gestation. An early pregnancy scan is suggestive of a molar pregnancy, and no fetus is observed.

   What is the typical genotype of a complete molar pregnancy?

   A 45 XO
   B 46 XX
   C 46 XXX
   D 69 XXY
   E 92 XXXY

3. A 50-year-old woman is admitted to hospital following a myocardial infarction. She remains hypotensive for several days. Her serum lactate becomes elevated and her serum urea nitrogen and creatinine are also increased. Microscopic urinalysis reveals granular and hyaline casts.

   Which of the following renal pathologies is most likely to be the cause?

   A Acute tubular necrosis
   B Chronic pyelonephritis
   C Minimal change glomerulonephritis
   D Nodular glomerulosclerosis
   E Renal vein thrombosis

4. A 43-year-old woman was diagnosed at 15 years of age with type 1 diabetes mellitus. Her disease has been poorly controlled. She developed a non-healing ulcer of her foot at 35 years of age. By 40 years of age, she had an increasing serum urea and a urinalysis shows a specific gravity of 1.012, pH 6.5, 1+ protein, no blood, 1+ glucose, negative leucocyte esterase, negative nitrite, and no ketones.

    Which of the following renal diseases is she most likely to have?

    A Crescentic glomerulonephritis
    B Hyperplastic arteriolosclerosis
    C Nodular glomerulosclerosis
    D Papillary necrosis
    E Pyelonephritis

5. A 59-year-old man presents with a 1-week history of frank haematuria. On physical examination, there are no abnormal findings. Urinalysis confirms the presence of blood, but no proteinuria or glycosuria. Urine culture is negative. A cystoscopy is performed, and a 3-cm exophytic mass is seen in the dome of the bladder. A biopsy of this mass is performed and microscopic examination reveals fibrovascular cores covered by a thick layer of transitional cells.

    Which of the following risk factors is most likely to have led to development of this lesion?

    A Chronic use of nonsteroidal anti-inflammatory drugs
    B Cigarette smoking
    C Diabetes mellitus
    D Recurrent urinary tract infection
    E Obesity

6. A 30-year-old woman has had increasing malaise with fever, abdominal pain, and weight loss of 3 kg over the past 3 weeks. On physical examination, her blood pressure is 160/110 mmHg. She has a stool positive for occult blood. Urinalysis reveals haematuria. She has no serum anti-neutrophil cytoplasmic autoantibodies and her antinuclear antibody test is negative. Aneurysmal arterial dilations and occlusions are seen in the medium-sized renal and mesenteric arteries with angiography. She improves with corticosteroid therapy.

    Which of the following is the most likely diagnosis?

    A Benign nephrosclerosis
    B Nodular glomerulosclerosis
    C Polyarteritis nodosa
    D Systemic lupus erythematosus
    E Wegener granulomatosis

7. A 55-year-old woman is admitted to the emergency department 1 week after a work-related crush injury. On physical examination, she is febrile and appears dehydrated. After catheterisation, she passes a small amount of very dark urine. The urine dipstick test for blood is positive but no red blood cells are seen on microscopy.

Her serum biochemistry shows:

Creatinine = 120 µmol/L

Serum potassium = 5.7 mmol/L

Creatinine kinase = >50,000 U/L

Which of the following is the most likely diagnosis?

A   Post-streptococcal glomerulonephritis
B   Renal infarction
C   Renal papillary necrosis
D   Rhabdomyolysis
E   Ureteral lithiasis

8. Which of the following is characteristic of the cellular changes seen in dysplasia?

A   Absence of mitotic figures on microscopy
B   Decreased mitotic activity
C   Hyperchromatism
D   Irreversibility
E   Uniformity in cell shape

9. Which of the following vulval skin disorders is associated with the highest risk of developing malignant disease?

A   Contact irritant dermatitis
B   Lichen planus
C   Lichen sclerosis
D   Squamous cell hyperplasia
E   Psoriasis

10. A 75-year-old woman presents to her general practitioner (GP) with increasing abdominal girth, reduced appetite and increasing shortness of breath. Her GP, suspicious of malignancy, performs laboratory investigations and refers her for an urgent review to the local hospital.

The results of her laboratory investigations are as follows:

Tumour marker	Result	Reference range
CA 19-9 (U/mL)	34	0–40
CA-125 (U/mL)	812	0–35
Carcinoembryonic antigen (µg/L)	1.2	0–2.5
A-Fetoprotein U/mL	1.4	0–5

From the tumour marker levels given, what is the most likely primary tumour?

A   Colorectal cancer
B   Hepatocellular cancer
C   Lung cancer with abdominal metastases

    D Pancreatic cancer
    E Primary peritoneal cancer

11. Which of the following paraneoplastic syndromes is paired with a recognised causal malignancy?

    A Acanthosis nigricans and bowel cancer
    B Carcinoid and uterine cancer
    C Cushing's syndrome and small cell lung cancer
    D Dermatomyositis and renal cancer
    E Syndrome of inappropriate antidiuretic hormone secretion and fibroma

12. Which of the following is a risk factor for the development of ovarian cancer?

    A Early menopause
    B History of breastfeeding
    C Nulliparity
    D Oral contraceptive use
    E Physical activity

13. A grand multiparous woman has a postpartum haemorrhage soon after delivery. She is tachycardic, hypotensive, with a capillary refill time of 3 seconds and she appears confused. She has grade IV haemorrhagic shock.

What do you think is the estimated blood loss thus far based on clinical findings?

    A 500 mL
    B 750 mL
    C 1000 mL
    D 1300 mL
    E 2000 mL

14. A 39-year-old woman has a forceps delivery. She is diagnosed as having a fourth degree tear of the perineum, which is repaired in theatre. She is readmitted 5 days later with wound dehiscence and it is noted that faecal matter is draining per vaginam. She has a temperature, is tachycardic and is feeling unwell. She is in septic shock soon after arrival.

Which of the below pathogens is the most likely causative agent?

    A *Actinomyces israelii*
    B *Clostridium perfringens*
    C *Staphylococcus aureus*
    D *Listeria monocytogenes*
    E *Escherichia coli*

Answers

1. A Breech presentation

A bicornuate uterus has an incidence of 0.1–0.5%. It is caused when the Müllerian (paramesonephric) ducts incompletely fuse during embryonic development. This results in two separate, but communicating, endometrial cavities. The extent to which there is incomplete fusion of the Mullerian ducts can result in varying degrees of abnormality. This varies from uterus didelphus where there are two entirely separate uterine cavities and a septate uterus where there is essentially a single uterine cavity interrupted by a thin septum. The presence of a bicornuate uterus is associated with recurrent miscarriage, breech presentation and preterm delivery. **Figure 13.1** shows different structural abnormalities of the uterus.

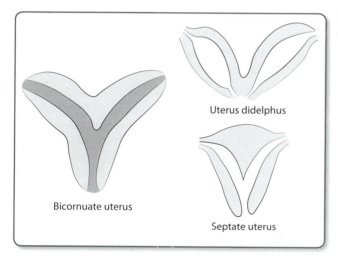

Figure 13.1 Structural abnormalities of the uterus.

Uterus didelphus

Bicornuate uterus

Septate uterus

2. B 46 XX

Gestational trophoblastic disease describes a variety of conditions ranging from complete and partial molar pregnancies to malignant choriocarcinoma. Histologically there is cystic swelling of chorionic villi.

A single sperm combining with an egg, which is devoid of DNA, usually causes a complete molar pregnancy. The genotype is usually diploid 46 XX, as a result of mitosis of the fertilising sperm. Occasionally the genotype is 46 XY.

Two sperm or one, which duplicates and has a triploid genotype 69 XXY, or quadraploid XXXY usually, causes a partial molar pregnancy. Gestational trophoblastic disease is a premalignant condition. Overall approximately 1–2% of hydatiform pregnancies develop into choriocarcinoma and complete moles are more likely to do so. They are diagnosed histologically by cystic swelling of chorionic villi and marked trophoblastic proliferation.

3. A Acute tubular necrosis

Acute tubular necrosis (ATN) is the commonest cause of acute renal failure, and is a renal cause (as opposed to pre-renal and post-renal causes). Acute tubular necrosis can be caused by a variety of insults including ischaemia, infection, toxins and drugs. Typically, ATN is characterised by injury to the tubular epithelial cells of the renal parenchyma leading to necrotic lesions and the formation of epithelial casts. Initially, ATN may present with a slightly reduced urine output, followed by profound oliguria, metabolic acidosis, uraemia and hyperkalaemia. When recovery begins there is a polyuria and an associated osmotic diuresis. If appropriately managed (i.e. using dialysis if needed), ATN can be reversible and there can be complete recovery if the cause is removed.

4. C Nodular glomerulosclerosis

Nodular glomerulosclerosis, also known as diabetic nephropathy, is a common complication of diabetes mellitus. The disease is characterised by thickening of the glomerulus basement membrane, mesangial sclerosis and glomerulosclerosis. These features are the sequelae of the known end-organ damage associated with diabetes mellitus as a consequence of microvascular disease and chronic hyperglycaemia.

This form of nephropathy is typically diagnosed in individuals with known diabetes mellitus, non-healing ulcers, proteinuria and retinopathy. The diagnosis is characterised by a progressively declining glomerular filtration rate, long-standing albuminuria and hypertension. The mainstay of treatment is improved glycaemic control, management of hypertension (often with the use of ACE inhibitors), dietary protein restriction and in some cases renal dialysis.

5. B Cigarette smoking

Cigarette smoking is known to be the greatest risk factor for the development of bladder cancer, and is thought to be associated with around 50% of cases. The disease is also more common in individuals who have worked in industrial settings and been exposed to carcinogens, such as aniline dyes. Exposure to cyclophosphamide is a further risk factor. An exophytic mass is a lesion that grows out of the surface of an organ. In this patient the mass represents a transitional cell carcinoma of the bladder. The patient has frank haematuria, which is the most common presenting symptom of this tumour of the urothelium. Management strategies of transitional cell carcinoma of this kind include bladder resection, cystectomy, chemotherapy and radiotherapy.

6. C Polyarteritis nodosa

Polyarteritis nodosa (PAN) is a systemic vasculitis of unknown aetiology, which affects the small and medium-sized arteries. Necrotising transmural inflammation is typical in affected vessels. There is associated microaneurysm formation, tissue infarction and necrosis. Lesions can affect the gastrointestinal tract, the kidneys, the heart and the liver. There may be resultant hypertension due to renal involvement, melaena due to gastrointestinal lesions alongside abdominal pain, malaise, fever and weight loss. PAN affects men more than women and typically presents in young adulthood. Diagnosis is usually made by renal biopsy or by mesenteric angiography. Although the aetiology of PAN is uncertain there appears to be an association with chronic hepatitis B infection, with around 30% of individuals with PAN having hepatitis B antibody complexes present in affected arteries. Corticosteroids and cyclophosphamide form the mainstay of treatment.

7. D Rhabdomyolysis

This woman's urinalysis shows myoglobinuria, which typically follows significant trauma to muscle tissue. Although its presence may have minimal sequelae in severe cases, there may be rhabdomyolysis. Myoglobin is normally renally-excreted, but in excessive amounts it causes obstruction of the distal tubule and acute renal failure. In rhabdomyolysis there is excessive release of the intracellular contents of muscle cells leading to hyperkalaemia and metabolic acidosis. Hypocalcaemia may also occur. In severe cases there may be disseminated intravascular coagulation.

8. C Hyperchromatism

Dysplasia is a term used to describe abnormal development of immature cells in a tissue, whereby there are abnormalities in the cellular architecture and appearance. Dysplastic cells can be thought of as showing some cellular changes that occur in cancer cells. These atypical features infer malignant potential although not all dysplastic tissue will go on to become malignant. In dysplastic cells a series of visible characteristic changes occur, which include:

- Increased mitotic activity
- Hyperchromatism: prominent cell nucleus due to increased chromatin
- Nuclear pleomorphism: abnormalities in the shape and size of the nucleus
- Anisocytosis: increased cell size
- Poikilocytosis: unusually shaped cells

Dysplasia may be reversible when in its early stages, especially if any causative stimulus can be removed. A potentially reversible form of dysplasia is present in CIN I, where dysplastic changes are only seen in the basal third of the squamous epithelium; in these cases there is high likelihood of reversible changes and monitoring may be appropriate.

9. C Lichen sclerosis

All options given are non-neoplastic skin conditions of the vulva. Vulval cancer is a rare form of cancer (1.7/100,000 women) usually affecting women around 70–80 years old; the majority of cases are squamous carcinomas (90%). Risk factors for the development of vulval cancer include: smoking, chronic skin conditions such as lichen sclerosis, vulval intraepithelial neoplasia (VIN), Paget's disease and the presence of melanoma in situ.

Lichen sclerosis is an inflammatory condition affecting the anogenital area; the majority of sufferers are postmenopausal women. Patients often present with itching. Treatments include use of potent topical corticosteroids. 5–7% of women may go on to develop vulval cancer. Vulval cancer spreads by direct extension to surrounding structures, local lymph nodes and by the blood stream.

10. E Primary peritoneal cancer

Primary peritoneal cancer (PPC), like ovarian cancer, is associated with high serum levels of the tumour marker CA-125. PPC is a rare cancer of the peritoneum. Like ovarian cancer, many patients have few symptoms until relatively late in the disease's progression. Invasion to the peritoneum is not uncommon in ovarian cancer, however there is often minimal or no ovarian involvement when there is a primary peritoneal cancer. PPC has an association with transmission of the oncogene BRCA1 and BRCA2. Treatment of PPC, like ovarian cancer, includes surgical interventions such as total abdominal hysterectomy, bilateral oophorectomy and omentectomy, as well as chemotherapy and radiotherapy. It is important to remember that whilst tumour markers can aid diagnosis they are limited in their specificity and sensitivity; they are especially useful for monitoring disease progression pre- and post-treatment (**Table 13.1**).

Table 13.1 Tumour markers and associated malignancies	
Tumour markers	**Associated malignancies**
CA 19-9	Colorectal cancer
	Pancreatic cancer
CA-125	Ovarian cancer
	Primary peritoneal cancer
CA 15-3	Breast cancer
Carcinogenic embryonic antigen	Colorectal cancer
Alpha-fetoprotein	Pancreatic cancer
	Germ cell tumours
Human chorionic gonadotrophin	Gestational trophoblastic disease
	Germ cell tumours
Prostate specific antigen	Prostate cancer

11. C Cushing's syndrome and small cell lung cancer

Paraneoplastic syndromes are groups of symptoms, which may present in patients with malignancy; the tumour itself does not directly cause them. Paraneoplastic syndromes may present as pathologies of the endocrinological, dermatological, rheumatological, haematological, renal, gastrointestinal and neuromuscular systems (**Table 13.2**).

Table 13.2 Paraneoplastic syndromes and their associated malignancies		
System	Paraneoplastic syndrome	Associated malignancies
Endocrine	Syndrome of inappropriate antidiuretic hormone secretion	Lung cancer Tumours of central nervous system
	Cushing's syndrome	Small cell lung cancer
Dermatological	Acanthosis nigricans	Uterine cancer
	Dermatomyositis	Breast cancer
Haematological	Polycythaemia	Renal cancer
	Lambert–Eaton myasthenic syndrome	Hepatocellular cancer Small cell lung cancer

12. C Nulliparity

There are a series of risk factors for ovarian cancer. The main risk factors for the development of ovarian cancer are increasing age, the presence of gene mutations such as BRCA and HNPCC and a family history of the disease. Several additional risk factors relate to ovarian activity, i.e. ovarian cancer appears to be less common in women who have interrupted ovulation during their reproductive years. The malignancy is more common in women who have an early menarche and a late menopause. Women who have had no pregnancies are at a greater risk of developing ovarian cancer; the more children a woman has had the lower the risk. Protective factors include those who have used the contraceptive pill and those with a history of breastfeeding.

13. E 2000 mL

This patient is obviously compromised by her blood loss and needs rapid fluid resuscitation and is likely also to need blood products. Haemorrhagic shock can be classified according to the amount of blood lost and the subsequent derangement in vital signs as the body tries to compensate for the blood loss. In addition to tachycardia, hypotension and tachypnoea, there may be altered consciousness and reduced urine output reflecting reduced organ perfusion. This patient's condition is suggestive a massive loss of blood volume, equivalent to around 2000 mL. This is classified as class IV haemorrhagic shock:

- Class I haemorrhage: up to 15% blood volume, up to around 750 mL blood loss
- Class II haemorrhage: 15–30% blood volume lost
- Class III haemorrhage: 30–40% blood volume lost
- Class IV haemorrhage: over 40% blood volume lost

14. E *Escherichia coli*

Most cases of septic shock are caused by infection with Gram-negative bacteria, although Gram-positive bacterium, viruses and fungi can be causative agents.

E. coli is the only Gram-negative bacterium of the options given and therefore the most likely cause of this patient's life-threatening condition. Gram-negative bacilli release endotoxins, which are bacterial wall lipopolysaccharides (LPS). LPS can lead to the systemic activation of macrophages, neutrophils, natural killer cells and the widespread release of cytokines and inflammatory mediators such as tumour necrosis factor and interleukins. The consequences of this immune system activation include vasodilation, increased vascular permeability and endothelial injury. Inflammatory mediators may activate the coagulation system leading to deranged clotting and in extreme cases disseminated intravascular coagulation. Untreated, septic shock may lead to death.

Chapter 14

Pharmacology

Questions

For each question, select the single best answer from the five options listed.

1. Which of the following normal physiological changes seen in pregnancy are associated with a slower drug metabolism?

    A   Delayed gastric emptying
    B   Increased body fat volume
    C   Increased cardiac output
    D   Increased glomerular filtration rate
    E   Increased third space volume

2. A 17-year-old girl discovers she is pregnant despite taking the oral contraceptive pill. She has recently been prescribed a new medication by her general practitioner.

    Which of the following drugs is most likely to have interacted with the efficacy of her contraception?

    A   Carbamazepine
    B   Cimetidine
    C   Erythromycin
    D   Metronidazole
    E   Sulphamethoxazole

3. Which of the following forms part of phase 2 reactions in drug metabolism?

    A   Conjugation
    B   Cyclisation
    C   Hydrolysis
    D   Reduction
    E   Oxidation

4. A 23-year-old woman is admitted to hospital as she is acutely unwell, having admitted to taking an overdose. On examination, her temperature is 38.6°C, blood pressure 105/68 mmHg, heart rate 96 beats per minute and a respiratory rate of 12 breaths per minute. Her arterial blood gas test shows respiratory alkalosis.

    What is the most likely drug overdose?

A   Amitriptyline
B   Aspirin
C   Cocaine
D   Tramadol
E   Zopiclone

5. A 27-year-old woman attends antenatal clinic at 14 weeks' gestation. This is her second pregnancy, and she suffered a pulmonary embolism during her first pregnancy 3 years ago. Her thrombophilia screen, taken prior to pregnancy, is negative.

What is the most appropriate course of action at this point?

A   Monitor closely for signs of thromboembolic event
B   Start prophylactic dose low-molecular weight heparin (LMWH) immediately
C   Start prophylactic dose LMWH at 24 weeks' gestation
D   Start treatment dose LMWH at 24 weeks' gestation
E   Urgent referral to haematology department

6. Which of the following is a recognised side effect of heparin usage?

A   Hirsutism
B   Hyperaldosteronism
C   Hypokalaemia
D   Osteomalacia
E   Thrombocytopaenia

7. A 37-year old-woman is requesting analgesia following a caesarean section. You notice that she has von Willebrand disease and wonder how this may affect her coagulation profile.

Which of the following set of blood tests is most likely to represent a patient with von Willebrand disease?

	Prothrombin time	Activated partial thromboplastin time	Bleeding time	Platelet count
A	Unaffected	Prolonged	Prolonged	Unaffected
B	Unaffected	Prolonged	Unaffected	Unaffected
C	Prolonged	Mildly prolonged	Unaffected	Unaffected
D	Prolonged	Prolonged	Prolonged	Decreased
E	Unaffected	Unaffected	Prolonged	Decreased

8. A 32-year-old woman suffers a 1500 mL postpartum haemorrhage 15 minutes after delivery. She is given several drugs to contract the uterus and the bleeding stops. One hour later, she is found to have blood pressure of 178/110 mmHg.

Which drug is most likely to be responsible for this clinical finding?

    A   Carboprost
    B   Ergometrine
    C   Misoprostol
    D   Oxytocin
    E   Ritodrine

9. A 2-year-old child has been investigated by the ear, nose and throat specialists for sensorineural hearing loss. Following a series of investigations he is found to have a defect of the 8th cranial nerve.

Which of the following medications did his mother take during her pregnancy?

    A   Chloramphenicol
    B   Co-trimoxazole
    C   Doxycycline
    D   Erythromycin
    E   Streptomycin

10. A 27-year-old woman is treated for severe bronchitis at 38 weeks' gestation. Her baby, born at 41 weeks' gestation, has neonatal haemolysis.

Which drug taken by the mother for bronchitis is the cause of the baby's neonatal haemolysis?

    A   Chloramphenicol
    B   Co-trimoxazole
    C   Doxycycline
    D   Erythromycin
    E   Streptomycin

11. A 35-year-old woman, with a history of previous multiple pulmonary embolisms, is now 8 weeks pregnant.

Which is the anticoagulant of choice during her pregnancy?

    A   Aspirin 300 mg
    B   Heparin infusion
    C   Low-molecular weight heparin
    D   Warfarin
    E   None of the above

12. A 25-year-old nulliparous woman, with a lifelong history of tonic-clonic seizures, sees her neurologist as she wishes to start a family.

In addition to her current anticonvulsant therapy which additional drug is now required?

    A   A second anticonvulsant
    B   Ferrous sulphate
    C   Folic acid
    D   Low-molecular weight heparin
    E   Vitamin K

13. A 23-year-old woman is 8 weeks pregnant. She has persistent itchy, thick, white vaginal discharge. A high vaginal swab has identified the presence of yeast species. She has already tried topical clotrimazole cream which has provided no relief of her symptoms.

   Which is the most appropriate treatment for vaginal candidiasis unresponsive to clotrimazole cream?

   A   Clotrimazole pessary
   B   Metronidazole 400 mg orally
   C   Fluconazole 400 mg orally
   D   Hydrocortisone 0.5% cream
   E   Trimovate creams

14. A female patient with well-controlled epilepsy attends clinic for some pre-conception advice.

   Which anti-epileptic drug carries the greatest risk of neural tube defects?

   A   Carbamazepine
   B   Lamotrigine
   C   Sodium valproate
   D   Phenytoin
   E   Tiagabine

15. A woman attends her GP surgery at 39 weeks' gestation with symptoms of a urinary tract infection (UTI).

   Which antibiotic is associated with a risk of neonatal haemolysis?

   A   Cephalexin
   B   Ciprofloxacin
   C   Gentamicin
   D   Nitrofurantoin
   E   Trimethoprim

Answers

1. A Delayed gastric emptying

The natural physiological changes in pregnancy lead to a change in the pharmacokinetics of drugs. Pregnancy is associated with delayed gastric emptying, which subsequently increases the bioavailability of drugs that are slowly absorbed. Increased third space volume leads to a greater area of distribution and therefore a lower plasma concentration. An increase in renal blood flow means faster renal clearance. In pregnancy there is a reduction in circulating binding proteins including albumin, and this leads to an increase in free levels of drugs that are usually bound to albumin.

2. A Carbamazepine

Carbamazepine is an enzyme inducer. Drugs acting as enzyme inducers increase the action of the enzyme system and lead to increased metabolism and therefore clearance of the drug. In this case, the oral contraceptive pill has been less effective due to the co-administration of an enzyme inducer. Other enzyme inducers include rifampicin and ethanol. The rest of the drugs on this list are enzyme inhibitors. Enzyme inhibitors increase the concentration and availability of other drugs as they prevent their metabolism.

3. A Conjugation

The process of elimination of a drug from the body is an irreversible process and occurs via metabolism and excretion. Drug metabolism occurs via phase 1 and phase 2 reactions, which both normally take place in the liver. Phase 1 reactions include oxidation, reduction or hydrolysis, with the resulting products being more reactive. Phase 2 reactions generally involve conjugation, e.g. with amino acids, leading to inactivation of the drug. Some of the products are excreted in bile after the phase two reactions.

4. B Aspirin

A large dose of aspirin results in the uncoupling of oxidative phosphorylation, which leads to higher consumption of oxygen and increased carbon dioxide. The higher carbon dioxide results in stimulation of the respiratory centre, causing hyperventilation and a respiratory alkalosis. Higher doses of salicylates can cause respiratory depression and produce respiratory acidosis. Increased temperature may result from an increased respiratory rate. Aspirin is a non-steroidal anti-inflammatory, and in normal doses is an effective antipyretic and analgesic.

Overdose of amitriptyline can cause nausea and vomiting, but may also have more serious side effects such as cardiac arrhythmia, agitation and unconsciousness. Tramadol is an opioid and zopiclone is a benzodiazepine. Both of these medications would lead to respiratory depression, but are unlikely to lead to a respiratory alkalosis or hyperpyrexia.

5. B Start prophylactic dose low-molecular weight heparin (LMWH) immediately

Pulmonary embolism (PE) during pregnancy is responsible for the greatest number of maternal deaths in the UK (1.56/100,000 pregnancies). It is therefore essential that any women who are clinically at risk of developing PE in pregnancy be recommended appropriate prophylaxis. The Royal College of Obstetrics and Gynaecology guideline recommends that antenatal thromboprophylaxis with LMWH is offered if there is a personal history of VTE in one of the following categories: recurrent, unprovoked, oestrogen-related, pregnancy-related, or associated with significant risk factors such as a documented thrombophilia.

In this case, the most appropriate answer is to start low-molecular weight heparin immediately. It should be started from the first trimester, however in cases where this has been missed; prophylactic dose should be commenced immediately. This patient should also be referred urgently to haematology, but this is not the best answer.

Royal College of Obstetricians and Gynaecologists. Reducing the Risk of Venous Thromboembolism During Pregnancy and the Puerperium. Green-top Guideline 37a. London: RCOG 2015.

6. E Thrombocytopaenia

Heparin prevents coagulation via the activation of antithrombin III. Binding of heparin to the antithrombin III changes its conformation and thereby speeds up its rate of action. There are several potential side effects of heparin and these include:

- Bleeding; treated by stopping heparin therapy or administering protamine
- Thrombocytopaenia; may be caused by IgM or IgG antibodies against circulating platelets
- Hypoaldosteronism; may be associated with hyperkalaemia, rather than hypokalaemia
- Osteoporosis; usually associated with long-term therapy. The mechanism is unknown

7. A

A	Unaffected	Prolonged	Prolonged	Unaffected

B represents haemophilia, C represents warfarin, D represents disseminated intravascular coagulation while E represents thrombocytopaenia.

Von Willebrand's disease is a common inherited haemostatic disorder, with an incidence of 1 in 10,000. It has autosomal inheritance and is equally prevalent in males and females. There are several types of disease, the most common being type I which shows autosomal dominant inheritance. Von Willebrand's disease is a deficiency in von Willebrand's factor, a protein that brings platelets into contact with damaged subendothelium, causing platelet adhesion and is essential for normal clotting. Patients often present with an abnormality of bleeding, which may manifest with nosebleeds, abnormal menses or easy bruising. Females often present with menorrhagia. The overall platelet count is not affected. These patients should not be given non-steroidal anti-inflammatories due to the prolonged bleeding time. Clotting profile may demonstrate a raised activated Prothrombin time (APTT); however, the international normalised ratio and platelets are usually normal.

8. B Ergometrine

Ergometrine is an ergot alkaloid which increases basal tone of the uterus. It has most effect on the uterus if it is not properly contracted. It has an effect of vasoconstriction. Side effects include vomiting via stimulation of the chemoreceptor trigger zone. The other drugs listed also contract the uterus, but only ergometrine can cause a rise in blood pressure as a result of the vasoconstriction effect.

9. E Streptomycin

The aminoglycosides, such as gentamicin and streptomycin, are known to damage the 8th cranial nerve in the developing fetus and are ototoxic when given in the second and third trimesters. The greatest risk to the fetus occurs with streptomycin, which has been associated with an incidence of 8th cranial nerve damage of > 10%. Gentamicin may be required during pregnancy, e.g. in severe urinary tract infections and should be given cautiously if indicated. In addition to the risks to the fetus, the aminoglycosides are associated with both ototoxicity and nephrotoxicity in adults.

10. B Co-trimoxazole

Historically, sulphonamides such as sulfadiazine were thought to increase the risk of neonatal kernicterus via displacement of bilirubin from albumin binding sites; however, this is now thought to be an unsubstantiated concern. Both the sulphonamides and trimethoprim are thought to cause neonatal haemolysis and methaemoglobinaemia and therefore should be avoided in third trimester. Co-trimoxazole, a mixture of the sulphonamide sulphamethoxazole and trimethoprim, is therefore to be avoided in pregnancy. In addition to the risks associated with the administration of these antimicrobials in the third trimester, trimethoprim is known to be teratogenic during the first trimester of pregnancy due to its action as a folate antagonist.

11. C Low-molecular weight heparin

Appropriate anticoagulation in pregnancy is determined by gestation. Warfarin is teratogenic and should be stopped before 6 weeks' gestation; heparin does not cross the placenta and therefore in its low-molecular weight form is an appropriate alternative to warfarin. Warfarin is present in breast milk, however not at levels known to be harmful, whereas heparin is not excreted in breast milk. Aspirin is an antiplatelet medication, which should be avoided, in the third trimester.

12. C Folic acid

All anticonvulsant drugs are associated with an increased risk of teratogenesis. This is thought to be due to their known inhibition of folate which is an essential cofactor involved in DNA synthesis.

Although neural tube defects are the most well-known malformations associated with the use of anticonvulsants, other problems such as cardiac defects, orofacial clefts and fetal anticonvulsant syndrome have been reported. Higher dose folic acid (5 mg daily) supplementation is required for those women using anticonvulsants in pregnancy and ideally should be started prior to conception in order to reduce the risk of malformations, such as neural tube defects, associated with lowered serum folate levels. Vitamin K should be given to the neonate to prevent the increased risk of haemorrhage associated with anticonvulsants. A second form of anticonvulsant therapy should only be commenced with caution as the risk of teratogenesis increases with the number of anticonvulsants used.

13. A Clotrimazole pessary

The yeast *Candida albicans* in most cases causes candidiasis. It is carried on the skin and in the gut. Vaginal candidiasis is common in pregnancy and this is partly due to the raised levels of oestrogen and a relative immunosuppressed state. It usually presents with vaginal itching and soreness and may be a recurrent infection. Diagnosis is confirmed by microscopy and culture of vaginal discharge. If a woman is asymptomatic with growth of *Candida* then there is no indication to treat the yeast. Symptomatic vaginal candidiasis may respond to clotrimazole in a pessary or cream form. Although used for resistant cases in non-pregnant women, oral antifungals should be avoided in pregnancy; fluconazole is known to cause congenital abnormalities when given at high doses over long periods.

14. C Sodium valproate

Epileptic patients have double the seizure risk during pregnancy. If the patient has been fit-free for 2 years, the risk of recurrent seizures whilst off medication is less than 20%. Pre-pregnancy counselling and optimisation of anti-epileptic medications should be arranged. If a woman is on any anti-epileptic agent they should take 5 mg of folic acid daily.

Of the anti-epileptics, sodium valproate is associated with the greatest risk of fetal developmental delay and neural tube defects. Phenytoin carries a high risk of facial cleft as it lowers serum folate levels. Carbamazepine is considered the safest anti-epileptic agent, and is associated with a risk of neural tube defects of less than 1%.

15. D Nitrofurantoin

Nitrofurantoin is avoided in the third trimester of pregnancy as there is an associated risk of neonatal haemolysis. Nitrofurantoin reduces activity of the enzyme glutathione reductase and this can lead to haemolytic anaemia in the newborn if the drug is given close to time of delivery.

Likely safe	Penicillins – 70% will cross the placenta, so can be used to treat fetal infection, e.g. syphilis
	Cephalosporins, e.g. cephalexin/ceftriaxone
	Macrolides e.g. Azithromycin/Erythromycin
Risk versus Benefit	Aminoglycosides, e.g. gentamicin/amikacin – risk of nephrotoxicity and 8th nerve damage
	Quinolones, e.g. ciprofloxacin – risk of arthropathy
	Nitrofurantoin – risk of neonatal haemolysis
	Chloramphenicol – grey baby syndrome and risk of cardiovascular collapse with systemic use
Avoid	Tetracyclines – permanent bone/teeth discolouration and impaired bone growth
	Sulphonamides, e.g. sulfadiazine (+ furosemide/gliclazide) – inhibit folate metabolism, Stevens–Johnson syndrome (allergy-toxic epidermal necrolysis), neonatal kernicterus

Chapter 15

Mock Paper 1

There are 100 single best answer (SBA) questions in this paper. The paper should be sat in exam conditions and completed in two and a half hours.

Questions

For each question, select the single best answer from the five options listed.

1. Which of the following structures does not pass through the diaphragm?

   A Azygos vein
   B Cisterna chyli
   C Inferior vena cava
   D Oesophagus
   E Thoracic duct

2. Which vessel provides blood supply to the intestine from the splenic flexure of the transverse colon to the rectum?

   A Inferior mesenteric artery
   B Median sacral artery
   C Middle colic artery
   D Rectal artery
   E Superior mesenteric artery

3. A 21-year-old woman undergoes a laparoscopic ovarian cystectomy to remove a dermoid cyst. The evening after the operation, she presents to the emergency department feeling unwell and her haemoglobin level is found to be 60 g/L. Damage to a blood vessel is suspected from the laparoscopic procedure.

   Which vessel crosses the common and external iliac artery in the infundibulopelvic fold?

   A Femoral artery
   B Inferior mesenteric artery
   C Median sacral artery
   D Ovarian artery
   E Renal artery

4. What is the nerve root of the ilioinguinal nerve?

    A T12 and L1
    B L1
    C L1 and L2
    D L2
    E L2 and L3

5. A 27-year-old woman has a cervical smear result, which shows 'borderline' changes.

    Which cells line the ectocervix?

    A Ciliated cells
    B Columnar epithelium
    C Cuboidal epithelium
    D Smooth muscle cells
    E Stratified squamous epithelium

6. A 32-year-old woman undergoes an emergency caesarean section for failure to progress at 9 cm cervical dilatation.

    Which of the following correctly describes the pelvic shape, which has an anteroposterior diameter of the inlet, greater than the transverse diameter?

    A Android
    B Anthropoid
    C Gynaecoid
    D Male
    E Platypelloid

7. An 18-year-old woman attends the gynaecology clinic complaining of urinary incontinence, 3 months after suffering a third degree perineal tear during a normal vaginal delivery.

    Which muscle forms the main bulk of the levator ani muscle?

    A Bulbocavernosus
    B Iliococcygeus
    C Ischiococcygeus
    D Pubococcygeus
    E Urogenital diaphragm

8. Which of the following organs is derived from ectodermal neural crest cells?

    A Adrenal gland inner medulla
    B Adrenal gland outer cortex
    C Liver
    D Pancreas
    E Spleen

9. A 63-year-old woman complains of numbness over her thigh following a radical hysterectomy for stage IV endometrial carcinoma.

   What is the nerve root of the obturator nerve?

   A   Anterior division L1–L4
   B   Anterior division L2–L4
   C   Anterior division L3–L4
   D   Posterior division L2–L4
   E   Posterior division L3–L4

10. What is the mechanism by which glucose crosses the placenta?

    A   Active transport
    B   Facilitated diffusion
    C   Immunoglobulin-binding proteins
    D   Osmosis
    E   Simple diffusion

11. A 38-year-old pregnant woman presents to the clinic complaining of epigastric pain at 34 weeks' gestation. Her liver function tests revealed high alanine transaminase (ALT), alkaline phosphatase (ALP) and bile acids.

    Other than from the bone and the liver, where is ALP produced?

    A   Fetus
    B   Gallbladder
    C   Ovary
    D   Placenta
    E   Stomach

12. A previously well, obese, primiparous 38-year-old woman who is 20 weeks pregnant undergoes an oral glucose tolerance test. Her fasting glucose was 5.5. The 2-hour result revealed a glucose level of 9.0.

    What is the interpretation of this result?

    A   Borderline gestational diabetes
    B   Gestational diabetes
    C   Impaired glucose tolerance
    D   Normal
    E   Type 2 diabetes

13. Which of the following has the correct association regarding development of urogenital system?

    A   Genital fold – clitoris
    B   Genital tubercle – labia minora
    C   Ureteric bud – urinary bladder
    D   Mesonephric ducts – vagina
    E   Metanephros – kidney

14. Which of the following statements best describes the development of the cardiac system?

   A   Fetal circulation includes two umbilical veins
   B   The ligamentum venosum is a remnant of the umbilical vein
   C   The heart is developed from endodermal cells
   D   The cardinal vein runs into the sinus venosus
   E   Cardiac pulsations are visible from the 34th day after conception

15. Which of the following is not a derivative of the vitelline vein?

   A   Lower inferior vena cava
   B   Inferior mesenteric vein
   C   Superior mesenteric vein
   D   Portal vein
   E   Hepatic vein

16. Which of the following statements best describes the development of the urogenital system?

   A   Sex cords are developed from coelomic epithelium
   B   Sex differentiation is present 35 days after fertilisation
   C   Myometrial walls are present in the fetal uterus by the 5th month
   D   Reproductive organs are developed from paraxial mesoderm
   E   In female sex organ development, the upper part of the gubernaculum becomes the round ligament

17. A 16-year-old girl is seen in the gynaecology outpatient department with primary amenorrhoea and excessive facial hair growth. Examination reveals normal genitalia, apart from an apparently large clitoris. Differential diagnosis includes congenital adrenal hyperplasia (CAH).

   CAH (21α-hydroxylase deficiency) is characterised by which of the following?

   A   Hypertension, hypokalaemia and hyponatraemia
   B   Hypertension, hyperkalaemia and hyponatraemia
   C   Hypotension, hyperkalaemia and hypernatraemia
   D   Hypotension, hyperkalaemia and hyponatraemia
   E   Hypotension, hypokalaemia and hyponatraemia

18. A 27-year-old woman is seen in the antenatal clinic. She suffered from hyperemesis gravidarum in the first trimester and routine thyroid function tests have revealed abnormalities.

   Which of the following is a recognised change in regulation of thyroid function in pregnancy?

   A   Decelerated T4 and T3 degradation and production rates
   B   Decreased basal metabolic rate
   C   Increased total T4 and T3 in the first trimester
   D   Increased thyroid-stimulating hormone
   E   Reduced plasma iodine concentration in early pregnancy

19. A 38-year-old woman is diagnosed with gestational diabetes requiring insulin treatment at 28 weeks' gestation.

Which of the following statements bests describes the function of human placental lactogen?

A It enhances amino acid transfer across the placenta
B It has insulin-like properties
C It increases glucose utilisation
D It increases insulin sensitivity in pregnancy
E It is a growth hormone antagonist

20. A 34-year-old woman is admitted to labour ward at 31 weeks' gestation with threatened preterm labour. As a precaution, she is given two doses of steroids.

Which of the following describes the first step in the synthesis of steroids?

A Conversion of cholesterol to pregnenolone
B Conversion of corticosterone to deoxycorticosterone
C Conversion of dehydroepiandrosterone to androstenedione
D Conversion of dihydrotesterone to oestradiol
E Conversion of pregnenolone to progesterone

21. Which of the following is an action of cortisol?

A Analgesic
B Decrease glycogenesis
C Decrease catabolism of proteins
D Decrease gastric acid production
E Increase gluconeogenesis

22. A 28-year-old woman is referred to the gynaecology clinic with primary infertility. On examination, she has a round face, prominent stretch marks on her abdomen and hirsuitism.

Which of the following is not a feature of Cushing's syndrome?

A Diabetes insipidus
B Depression
C Irregular menstrual cycles
D Osteoporosis
E Weight gain

23. A 26-year-old woman is referred to the gynaecology clinic with abdominal pain and amenorrhoea. You suspect she may have Cushing's syndrome and decide to send her for further tests.

Which of the following tests would be suitable for confirmation of the diagnosis?

A Adrenocorticotrophic hormone levels
B High dose dexamethasone suppression test
C Low-dose dexamethasone suppression test
D Short synacthen test
E Urinary free cortisol

24. A 52-year-old woman with Cushing's syndrome is referred to the pre-assessment clinic prior to a vaginal hysterectomy.

Which of the following is a feature of Cushing's syndrome?

A   Decreased plasma lactate dehydrogenase
B   Hypoglycaemia
C   Hypokalaemia
D   Hyponatraemia
E   Metabolic acidosis

25. An early pregnancy unit undertakes a study to look at the average serum β-human chorionic gonadotrophin (β-hCG) level of two hundred women presenting to their unit with vaginal spotting over a 2-month period.

The data collected has a normal distribution. The following values are obtained: mean = 500 IU/L, variance = 16.

What is the standard deviation of the dataset?

A   2
B   3
C   4
D   9
E   12

26. Which of the following is an aim of clinical audit?

A   To reject or accept a null hypothesis
B   To assess the extent to which current practice meets a defined set of standards
C   To assess differences between two different populations
D   To establish what is best practice
E   To extrapolate theory into practice

27. A study was designed to look at the relative risk of women with gestational diabetes mellitus (GDM) who delivered babies with a birth weight of over 4.5 kg. The study looked at all births in a maternity unit over a period of 1 year and classified whether the woman had GDM or not, and whether their baby weighed more or less than 4.5 kg.

Birth weight	Diabetic (n)	control (n)	Total
> 4.5 kg	80	50	130
< 4.5 kg	120	950	1070
Total	200	1000	1200

What is the relative risk of women with GDM delivering a baby weighing > 4.5 kg in this study?

A   0.05
B   0.1

    C   0.4
    D   8
    E   150

28. In therapeutic studies, what level of evidence is afforded to at least one well-designed controlled study without randomisation?

    A   1
    B   2a
    C   2b
    D   3
    E   4

29. Concerning chromosomes, which of the following statements is correct?

    A   Each consists of two identical chromatids
    B   They are best visualised during interphase
    C   The short arm of a chromosome is also known as the q arm
    D   Humans have 23 pairs of autosomal chromosomes
    E   The centromere lies at the distal end of the p arm

30. A 27-year-old woman attends the antenatal clinic at 16 weeks' gestation in her first pregnancy. Her brother suffers from cystic fibrosis and she did not have genetic counselling prior to conception, as this pregnancy was unplanned. She has some questions about cystic fibrosis.

Which of the following statements is correct?

    A   It is an X-linked recessive condition
    B   It is associated with gene defect of chromosome 9
    C   It is most commonly caused by deletion of F509
    D   It is characterised by a defect in potassium ion transport
    E   It is caused by a defect in the cystic fibrosis transmembrane conductance gene

31. Which of the following is caused by a microdeletion of chromosome 5?

    A   Angelman syndrome
    B   Cri-du-chat
    C   Di-George syndrome
    D   Rett syndrome
    E   Tay–Sachs disease

32. A couple are referred to geneticist for counselling as the woman's sister had a baby born with a chromosomal abnormality, thought to be Turner's syndrome.

Which of the following statements regarding aneuploidies is most accurate?

    A   Trisomy 16 is the most common trisomy in miscarried foetuses
    B   Monosomy X is incompatible with life
    C   Individuals with Triple X have multiorgan abnormalities
    D   Noonan's syndrome is caused by trisomy of chromosome 12
    E   The majority of trisomies follow a non-disjunction event at meiosis II

33. A 35-year-old woman at 30 weeks' gestation presents with an episode of vaginal spotting of fresh red blood. On speculum examination changes are noted to the vaginal portion of the cervix. There is also contact bleeding on taking a swab.

What is the histological change that occurs with a benign ectropion?

A Anaplasia
B Dysplasia
C Hyperplasia
D Metaplasia
E Neoplasia

34. A 30-year-old woman is diagnosed with polycystic ovarian syndrome (PCOS), according to the Rotterdam criteria. What are the typical hormonal changes associated with PCOS?

A High FSH:LH ratio, low SHBG
B High FSH:LH ratio, high SHBG
C Low FSH:LH ratio, low SHBG
D Low FSH:LH ratio, high SHBG
E Unchanged FSH:LH ratio, unchanged SHBG level

35. In the pregnant-state, what are the normal hormone changes of sex-hormone binding globulin (SHBG), oestradiol and cortisol, compared with non-pregnant state?

A High SHBG, high oestradiol, high progesterone
B High SHBG, low oestradiol, low progesterone
C Unchanged SHBG, high oestradiol, high progesterone
D Low SHBG, high oestradiol, low progesterone
E Low SHBG, low oestradiol, high progesterone

36. You are asked to review an arterial blood gas test (ABG) in a 32-year-old unwell pregnant woman who is at 32 weeks' gestation. The ABG shows a respiratory alkalosis with metabolic compensation.

Which part of the kidney is most responsible for the reabsorption of the bicarbonate ions?

A Collecting duct
B Distal tubule
C Loop of henle
D Nephron
E Proximal tubule

37. A post-menopausal woman presents with a low-impact fragility fracture of the femur.

What percentage of calcium in the body is stored within the skeletal system?

A 1%
B 10%

C 50%
D 90%
E 99%

38. A 29-year-old woman presents at 34 weeks' gestation with intense itching and is diagnosed with obstetric cholestasis.

What is the physiological need for bile salts?

A Absorption of amino acids
B Absorption of fats
C Conjugation of bilirubin
D No known physiological function
E Production of prostaglandins

39. A 29-year-old woman presents at 35 weeks' gestation with significant painful lower limb varicose veins.

What is the single most likely cause for worsening of varicose veins in pregnancy?

A Increased cardiac output
B Reduced vascular tone
C Pressure on the inferior vena cava
D Increased stroke volume
E Increased glomerular filtration rate

40. A 30-year-old woman presents at 30 weeks' gestation complaining of breathlessness.

What is the physiological change in tidal volume in pregnancy?

A Decreases by 30–40%
B Decreases by 70–80%
C No change
D Increases by 30–40%
E Increases by 70–80%

41. Which muscle lies within the rectus sheath and is supplied by the subcostal nerve?

A External oblique
B Internal oblique
C Pyramidalis
D Rectus abdominis
E Transversus abdominis

42. Which muscle enters the abdomen behind the medial arcuate ligament?

A External oblique
B Iliacus
C Psoas
D Pyramidalis
E Transversus abdominis

43. Which muscle forms part of the inguinal ligament?

    A   External oblique
    B   Iliacus
    C   Internal oblique
    D   Rectus abdominis
    E   Transversus abdominis

44. Which artery is the terminal branch of the internal thoracic artery?

    A   Inferior mesenteric artery
    B   Inferior phrenic artery
    C   Lumbar artery
    D   Superior epigastric artery
    E   Superior mesenteric artery

45. Which artery arises from the posterior trunk of the internal iliac artery?

    A   Inferior gluteal artery
    B   Middle rectal artery
    C   Superior gluteal artery
    D   Superior vesical artery
    E   Uterine artery

46. A 41-year-old woman complains of prolonged numbness in her leg 2 days after a normal vaginal delivery. She had an epidural for pain relief during labour.

What is the nerve root origin of lateral cutaneous nerve of the thigh?

    A   L1
    B   L2
    C   L3
    D   L1 and L2
    E   L2 and L3

47. A 25-year-old woman has a routine smear test for the first time. She complains of discomfort during the procedure.

Which nerve or nerve plexus carries afferent fibres from the cervix to the upper sacral nerves?

    A   Inferior hypogastric plexus
    B   Obturator nerve
    C   Pelvic splanchnic nerves
    D   Pudendal nerve
    E   Superior hypogastric plexus

48. A 72-year-old woman is referred to the gynaecology outpatient clinic with a 2-day history of postmenopausal bleeding. She subsequently undergoes a hysteroscopy and endometrial biopsy as part of her investigation.

Which of the following best describes the cells that line the uterus?

A   Columnar epithelium
B   Cuboidal epithelium
C   Pseudostratified columnar epithelium
D   Stratified squamous epithelium
E   Transitional cells

49. A 63-year-old woman is referred to the urogynaecology clinic with recurrent urinary tract infections and microscopic haematuria. A midstream urine sample is sent for cytology.

Which cells line the distal half of the urethra?

A   Columnar epithelium
B   Epidermis
C   Secretory cells
D   Stratified squamous epithelium
E   Transitional cells

50. An 82-year-old woman undergoes a vaginal hysterectomy for treatment of her procidentia. You are revising the stages of the operation.

Which ligament runs laterally from the body of the uterus, through the internal inguinal ring to the labium majus?

A   Broad ligament
B   Cardinal ligament
C   Iliolumbar ligament
D   Round ligament
E   Uterosacral ligament

51. Which of the following runs outside of the ischiorectal fossa?

A   Pudendal canal
B   Fat pad
C   Inferior rectal nerve
D   Middle rectal artery
E   Perineal branch of S4 nerve

52. Which of the following is correct regarding the embryological origin of the anal canal?

A   Above pectinate line: derived endoderm, superior rectal artery
B   Above pectinate line: derived ectoderm, superior rectal artery
C   Above pectinate line: derived ectoderm, columnar epithelium
D   Below pectinate line: derived ectoderm, superior rectal artery
E   Below pectinate line: derived endoderm, middle and inferior rectal artery

53. Prior to a forceps delivery, you wish to give a pudendal nerve block.

   Where is the pudendal canal?

   A   Lateral wall of ischiorectal fossa; above sacrotuberous ligament
   B   Lateral wall of ischiorectal fossa; below sacrospinous ligament
   C   Lateral wall of ischiorectal fossa; below sacrotuberous ligament
   D   Medial wall of ischiorectal fossa; above sacrospinous ligament
   E   Medial wall of ischiorectal fossa; below sacrotuberous ligament

54. A 24-year-old woman is catheterised prior to a diagnostic laparoscopy to investigate chronic pelvic pain.

   The distal aspect of the female urethra is lined with which type of epithelial cells?

   A   Ciliated
   B   Simple cuboidal
   C   Simple squamous
   D   Stratified squamous
   E   Transitional

55. A 26-year-old woman attends her general practitioner for her 6-week postnatal check. She has a central abdominal protrusion, which is diagnosed as a divarication of the rectus muscle.

   What is the nerve supply to the rectus abdominis muscle?

   A   T2–T12
   B   T7–T12
   C   T12–L3
   D   L2–L5
   E   L5–S3

56. A 32-year-old woman attends the gynaecology outpatient clinic complaining of severe premenstrual symptoms and pelvic pain. Her 4-year-old son is also present and it is noticed that he has an abnormal gait, with slightly bent and shortened legs.

   What is the most likely diagnosis of this child?

   A   Congenital abnormality
   B   Osteopetrosis
   C   Perthes disease
   D   Rickets
   E   Scurvy

57. A 65-year-old man attends his general practitioner with a 3-month history of lower backache and fatigue.

   Blood tests reveal the following:
   Urea   13.2 mmol/L
   Creatinine   145 µmol/L

Potassium	5.9 mmol/L
Haemoglobin	98 g/L
Mean corpuscular volume	82.2 fL/red cell
Calcium	2.65 mmol/L

What is the most likely diagnosis?

A Bone metastases
B Immobilisation
C Multiple myeloma
D Sarcoidosis
E Thiazide diuretics

58. A 62-year-old woman is diagnosed with a glucagonoma. Which one of the following metabolic conditions is most likely to result from this tumour?

A Decreased lipolysis
B Hyperglycaemia
C Increased muscle protein synthesis
D Increased liver glycolytic rate
E Increased glycogenesis

59. A 42-year-old woman is day 3 after a total abdominal hysterectomy for menorrhagia and fibroids. She is acutely short of breath, with pain on inspiration.

Her observations are as follows: Spo_2 93% on room air, blood pressure 115/74 mmHg, heart rate 105 beats per minute, respiratory rate 22 breaths per minute.

You perform an arterial blood gas. You are concerned she may have a pulmonary embolus. Considering this being the most likely diagnosis, which is the most likely result?

A pH 6.90, Pco_2 7.5 kPa, Po_2 15.1 kPa, HCO_3 15.4 mmol/L, base excess –12 mmol/L
B pH 7.16, Pco_2 8.2 kPa, Po_2 8.8 kPa, HCO_3 21.2 mmol/L
C pH 7.36, Pco_2 5.6 kPa, Po_2 13.2 kPa, HCO_3 26.0 mmol/L
D pH 7.50, Pco_2 3.0 kPa, Po_2 9.2 kPa, HCO_3 25.0 mmol/L
E pH 7.52, Pco_2 6.0 kPa, Po_2 12.0 kPa, HCO_3 17 mmol/L, base excess +4.5 mmol/L

60. A 28-year-old woman is admitted to the high dependency unit following a caesarean section. She was diagnosed during pregnancy with acute fatty liver of pregnancy. She was started on a morphine infusion postoperatively and is receiving oxygen by mask. She is noted to be very drowsy.

You perform an arterial blood gas. What is the most likely result in this case?

A pH 7.16, Pco_2 8.2 kPa, Po_2 15.3 kPa, HCO_3 21.2 mmol/L
B pH 7.20, Pco_2 4.8 kPa, Po_2 10.2 kPa, HCO_3 14 mmol/L
C pH 7.36, Pco_2 5.6 kPa, Po_2 13.2 kPa, HCO_3 26 mmol/L
D pH 7.52, Pco_2 6.0 kPa, Po_2 12.0 kPa, HCO_3 17 mmol/L
E pH 7.62, Pco_2 6.2 kPa, Po_2 12.2 kPa, HCO_3 15 mmol/L

61. A 23-year-old woman is admitted to hospital complaining of abdominal pain and vomiting. She is a type I diabetic and did not take her insulin today as she has been vomiting for 12 hours. On examination, she is tachycardic and feels cold and clammy.

An arterial blood gas confirms your diagnosis of ketoacidosis. Which of the following findings is most correct regarding diabetic ketoacidosis?

   A   High blood levels of fatty acids
   B   Hypoventilation
   C   Increased blood volume
   D   Low levels of lactate
   E   Respiratory acidosis

62. A 72-year-old woman is seen in the pre-assessment clinic prior to a hysteroscopy to investigate postmenopausal bleeding. She is taking aspirin and is asked to stop taking it 5 days prior to the procedure.

Which of the following prostanoids inhibits platelet aggregation?

   A   Prostacyclin PGI2
   B   Prostaglandin E2
   C   Prostaglandin D2
   D   Prostaglandin F2α
   E   Thromboxane TXA2

63. A 27-year-old woman is admitted to hospital with acute left iliac fossa pain, a positive pregnancy test and a haemoglobin level of 79 g/L. She undergoes a diagnostic laparoscopy and is found to have an ectopic pregnancy.

Where is the most common site of fertilisation of the ovum?

   A   Fimbria of the fallopian tube
   B   Ampulla of the fallopian tube
   C   Isthmus of the fallopian tube
   D   Tubal ostia
   E   Fundal endometrium

64. A 28-year-old woman is admitted to hospital with acute-onset right iliac fossa pain. She has low-grade pyrexia and is nauseous. Her blood tests reveal a C-reactive protein of 62 mg/dL and white cell count of 17.2×10^9/L. A diagnostic laparoscopy reveals a Meckel's diverticulitis.

Meckel's diverticulum is the persistence of which structure?

   A   Urachal remnant
   B   Vitellointestinal duct
   C   Primitive streak
   D   Paraxial mesoderm
   E   Buccopharyngeal membrane

65. Which one of the following is a derivative of the urogenital sinus in males?

A   Vas deferens
B   Epididymis
C   Ejaculatory duct
D   Prostate
E   Seminal vesicle

66. A 56-year-old woman attends her general practitioner's surgery complaining of feeling unwell for the last couple of months. The general practitioner decides to do a range of blood tests, including thyroid function, liver function and calcium and vitamin D levels.

Which of the following is associated with hypercalcaemia?

A   Chvostek's sign
B   Numbness
C   Perioral tingling
D   Shortened Q–T interval and widened T wave on ECG
E   Trousseau's sign

67. After an uneventful pregnancy a baby is born via spontaneous vaginal delivery. Soon after birth the midwife asks the paediatric team to review the baby, as she is uncertain of the infant's sex. Following a series of investigations the baby is found to have the genotype 46 XX and is diagnosed with congenital adrenal hyperplasia (CAH).

CAH is most commonly associated with a deficiency of which enzyme?

A   5α-reductase
B   11β-hydroxylase
C   17α-hydroxylase
D   21α-hydroxylase
E   Aromatase

68. A 26-year-old woman complains of increased facial hair and thinks it may be caused by a new medication she was prescribed 3 months previously.

Which of the following drugs is known to cause hirsutism?

A   Dianette
B   Erythromycin
C   Gentamicin
D   Phenytoin
E   Tacrolimus

69. Where is thyroid-stimulating hormone produced?

A   Acidophils of the anterior pituitary gland
B   Basophils of the anterior pituitary gland
C   Chromophobes of the anterior pituitary gland
D   Supraventricular nucleus of the hypothalamus
E   Paraventricular nucleus of the hypothalamus

70. Which of the following is a symptom of hyperthyroidism?

A Diarrhoea
B Infertility
C Palpitations
D Weight loss
E All of the above

71. The majority of extracellular calcium is bound to which of the following:

A Albumin
B Bicarbonate
C Calcitriol
D Fibrinogen
E Phosphate

72. A 63-year-old man attends his general practitioner with a 2-month history of lower back pain associated with radiation of pain down the right leg and shortness of breath. He has also lost some weight. Blood tests reveal: calcium 2.72 mmol/L, haemoglobin 104 g/L, mean corpuscular volume 83.6 L.

Which of the following is the most likely diagnosis?

A Bone metastases
B Immobilisation
C Osteoporosis
D Multiple myeloma
E Sarcoidosis

73. A junior doctor is asked to check the calcium levels on a patient 46 hours after a removal of her parathyroid gland.

Which of the following is a function of parathyroid hormone (PTH)?

A In bone, PTH reduces osteoclast activity
B PTH acts in the kidney to reduce bicarbonate excretion
C PTH acts on the kidney to increase level of phosphate absorption
D PTH acts to reduce serum levels of calcium
E PTH acts via a G-protein coupled receptor

74. Calcium is transferred from maternal circulation to fetal circulation via which transport mechanism?

A Active transport
B Endocytosis
C Exocytosis
D Facilitated diffusion
E Passive diffusion

75. Which of the following is true regarding maternal calcium homeostasis during pregnancy?

A   Increased calcitonin
B   Reduced 1,25 vitamin D3
C   Reduced bone turnover
D   Reduced calcium absorption
E   Increased parathyroid hormone production

76. Which of the following gives the World Health Organization's definition of neonatal mortality rate?

A   The number of deaths during the first 28 completed days of life per 1000 live births
B   The number of deaths during the first 28 completed days of life per 100,000 live births
C   The number of deaths during the first 365 completed days of life per 1000 live births
D   The number of deaths during the first 365 completed days of life per 10,000 live births
E   The number of deaths, including stillborn fetuses of more than 24 weeks' gestation, up to 28 completed days of life, per 1000 pregnancies

77. The quadruple test is a widely used screening test that aims to identify pregnancies with a high-risk of chromosomal abnormalities.

Which of the following gives the best definition of the test's specificity?

A   The proportion of women with a normal pregnancy who had a low-risk result
B   The proportion of women with an affected fetus who had a high-risk result
C   The proportion of women with a high-risk test result with an affected fetus
D   The proportion of women with a low-risk test result with a normal pregnancy
E   None of the above

78. The age of menarche was recorded for 100 women who attended a rapid access gynaecology clinic with suspected ovarian cancer. The data obtained showed a normal distribution. The mean age was 13 years and the standard deviation was 2 years.

What is the standard error of the mean for this sample?

A   0.1
B   0.2
C   0.5
D   1
E   2

79. A research study is designed to look at the association between mothers who smoke during pregnancy and the subsequent growth of their children. The study population is all babies born in the Maternity Unit between 1975 and 1980. The babies were classified at birth as having being born to women who smoked during their pregnancies or not. All of the children have their height and weight measured every year from birth to the age of 20 years.

What study design is being used?

A   Case-control study
B   Cohort study
C   Cross-sectional study
D   Double-blinded study
E   None of the above

80. Which of the following best describes a type 1 error?

A   The erroneous acceptance of the null hypothesis
B   The erroneous rejection of the null hypothesis
C   The inclusion of extreme outliers in a data set
D   The occurrence of a γ error
E   None of the above

81. Which of the following is a direct cause of maternal mortality?

A   Diabetes
B   Hormone-dependent breast cancer
C   Obesity
D   Community-acquired Group A streptococcal disease
E   Suicide

82. Which of following statements defines the median in a data set?

A   The least frequently occurring value in a data set
B   The middle value in a ranked set of data
C   The middle value in an unranked data set
D   The most frequently occurring value in a data set
E   The value obtained by dividing the sum of the data set by the number of values in the data set

83. A 28-year-old woman who is 13 weeks pregnant consents for routine antenatal screening. The results of her quadruple test show the fetus has a 1 in 58 chance of having trisomy 13.

What is trisomy 13 commonly known as?

A   Cri-du-chat syndrome
B   Down's syndrome
C   Edwards' syndrome
D   Patau's syndrome
E   Wolf–Hirschhorn syndrome

84. A 16-year-old boy's parents bring him the general practitioner. They are concerned that he appears to have developed breast tissue. On questioning, he feels self-conscious about his appearance and feels his genitalia are smaller than individuals of his own age. On examination, he appears tall for his age, with objectively long arms and legs. Gynaecomastia is noted, alongside a fat distribution typically seen in females.

What is the most likely genotype of this individual?

A   45 XO
B   46 XO
C   46 XX
D   46 XY
E   47 XXY

85. A 40-year-old primiparous woman has an elevated risk of trisomy 21 (1 in 50) at antenatal screening and opts for an amniocentesis at 15 weeks' gestation. The fetus is found to have the karyotype 46 XX/47 XX + 21.

What may this karyotype indicate?

A   Trisomy 21
B   Turner's syndrome
C   Klinefelter syndrome
D   Mosaic for Down's syndrome
E   None of above

86. A couple is seen for preconception counselling. The male is 26 years of age and of above-average height with noticeably long arms. He is being monitored for worsening aortic root dissection and has had pleurodesis for recurrent pneumothoraces. His vision is mildly impaired due to optic lens subluxation. The couple wishes to use preimplantation genetic screening techniques to prevent their children from inheriting their father's condition.

Which genetic condition does the male partner have?

A   Congenital contractual arachnodactyly
B   Ehlers–Danlos syndrome
C   Klinefelter syndrome
D   Marfan's syndrome
E   Triple X syndrome

87. Which of the following conditions is transmitted via mitochondrial inheritance?

A   Alpha-thalassaemia
B   Colour blindness
C   Dermatomyositis
D   Duchenne muscular dystrophy
E   Leber's optic neuropathy

88. Which of the following genetic conditions occurs as a result of genomic imprinting?

    A   Angelman's syndrome
    B   Fragile-X syndrome
    C   Friedreich ataxia
    D   Patau's syndrome
    E   All of the above

89. Which of the following hormones does the human placenta not secrete?

    A   Human chorionic gonadotrophin
    B   Oestrogen
    C   Oxytocin
    D   Progesterone
    E   Relaxin

90. At a term delivery, there is some concern about the placental structure. Which of the following statements about the umbilical cord is correct?

    A   At term the mean length is 70 cm
    B   It is formed at 8 weeks' gestation
    C   3% of cords have a single artery
    D   Umbilical arteries arise from the internal iliac artery
    E   Venous drainage is mainly to the inferior vena cava via the ductus arteriosus

91. Considering placental transport, which of the following are correctly paired?

    A   Active transport: amino acids
    B   Active transport: glucose
    C   Facilitated diffusion: free fatty acids
    D   Passive diffusion: glucose
    E   Receptor mediated endocytosis: IgA

92. Which of the following is a systemic function of oestrogen?

    A   Increases bone resorption
    B   Increases cholesterol levels
    C   Promotes atherosclerosis
    D   Vasoconstriction
    E   Vasodilation

93. A 22-year-old woman has undergone an evacuation of the retained products of conception (ERCP) after a missed miscarriage. The estimated blood loss was 1000 mL. You are called to see her, as she is hypotensive, and you wish to administer intravenous fluids.

Which of the following is correct regarding 0.9% sodium chloride?

    A   It contains 9 mmol/L sodium chloride
    B   It contains 154 mmol/L sodium chloride

C   It contains 18 mmol/L potassium chloride
D   It is a better volume expander than Hartmann's solution
E   It is the first choice of fluid in the immediate postoperative period

94. Which of the following statements is correct in regard to the double Bohr effect?

A   The fetal side becomes acidotic
B   The fetus loses metabolites to the mother
C   Maternal and fetal oxygen dissociation curves move towards each other
D   The maternal oxygen dissociation curve shifts to the left
E   The maternal side has an increased pH

95. What is the structure of fetal haemoglobin?

A   Two alpha chains and two beta chains ($\alpha2\beta2$)
B   Two alpha chains and two delta chains ($\alpha2d2$)
C   Two alpha chains and two gamma chains ($\alpha2\gamma2$)
D   Two beta and two delta chains ($\beta2d2$)
E   Two beta and two gamma chains ($\beta2\gamma2$)

96. A 21-year-old woman is seen in the gynaecology clinic complaining of pain in the lower abdomen during the middle of her menstrual cycle.

A surge in which hormone around day 14 of the menstrual cycle leads to ovulation?

A   Follicle-stimulating hormone
B   Luteinising hormone
C   Oestradiol
D   Progesterone
E   Testosterone

97. During oogenesis, at what point is the second meiotic division is completed?

A   At ovulation
B   Immediately prior to the formation of the secondary oocyte
C   Immediately prior to the formation of the primary oocyte
D   At fertilisation
E   None of the above

98. Which of the following structures communicates with the umbilical vein to form the ductus venosus?

A   Aorta
B   Inferior vena cava
C   Left atrium
D   Pulmonary artery

    E   Right atrium

99. Which of the following is a branch of the posterior division of the internal iliac artery?

    A   Inferior gluteal artery
    B   Internal pudendal artery
    C   Obturator artery
    D   Superior gluteal artery
    E   Uterine artery

100. After an elective caesarean section the anaesthetic team decide to administer a transversus abdominis plane block to provide analgesia. They use ultrasound to identify the layers of the abdominal wall.

Which of these muscles does the femoral nerve innervate?

    A   External oblique
    B   Iliacus
    C   Internal oblique
    D   Rectus abdominis
    E   Transverse abdominis

Answers

1. B Cisterna chyli

The cisterna chyli is a dilated sac at the base of the thoracic duct. It forms part of the lymphatic drainage from the pelvis and abdomen. The lymph passes to the thoracic duct that, after passing through the aortic hiatus, opens into the junction of the left subclavian vein and internal jugular vein.

2. A Inferior mesenteric artery

The inferior mesenteric artery arises just behind the horizontal part of duodenum (part 4). It lies retroperitoneally and crosses the left common iliac artery, medial to the ureter. The distribution of blood supply extends from the splenic flexure to the upper part of the rectum, which includes the descending colon and sigmoid colon. The distribution of the inferior mesenteric artery corresponds to the embryonic hindgut. Branches include the left colic artery and the superior rectal artery.

Table 15.1 Apertures of the diaphragm		
	Level	**Structure**
Caval opening	T8	Inferior vena cava
		Branches phrenic nerve
Oesophageal opening	T10	Oesophagus
Aortic hiatus	T12	Aorta
		Thoracic duct
		Azygos vein

3. D Ovarian artery

Ovarian arteries form branches of the abdominal aorta. They run retroperitoneally, leaving the abdomen by crossing the common or external iliac arteries in the infundibulopelvic fold. They are medial to the ureter in the upper abdomen and cross obliquely, anterior to the ureter in the middle to lower lumbar region, lying lateral to the ureter in the lower abdomen and pelvis. The infundibulopelvic ligament is a fold of the peritoneum, also known as the suspensory ligament of the ovary. It passes laterally from the ovary to the wall of the pelvis. See **Figure 15.1** for the abdominal aorta and its branches.

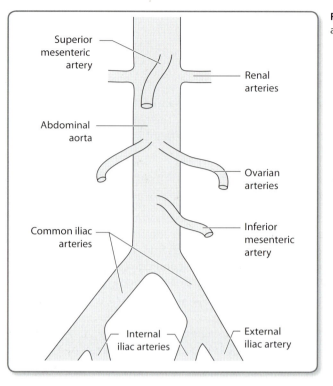

Figure 15.1 Abdominal aorta and its branches.

---

4. B L1

The ilioinguinal nerve arises from the L1 nerve root along with the larger iliohypogastric nerve. It travels obliquely across the quadratus lumborum and perforates the transversus abdominis near the anterior part of the iliac crest. It travels through part of the inguinal canal, passing through the superficial inguinal ring. It supplies the mons pubis and labium majus.

---

5. E Stratified squamous epithelium

The cervix has a conical shape with a varied epithelium. The ectocervix is the lower intravaginal portion of the cervix and is lined by non-keratinised stratified squamous epithelium. The endocervix is the cavity of the cervix, linking the external and the internal os. It is lined by mucin-secreting simple columnar epithelium. The border between these two types of epithelium is the squamocolumnar junction, or transformation zone. The transformation zone is the area where metaplasia frequently takes place and it is from here that the cervical smear test is taken. There are certain times when metaplasia is physiological, such as during puberty when the endocervix everts and postmenopause when the transformation zone moves upwards.

6. B Anthropoid

The basic shapes of the pelvis are as follows:

- Gynaecoid pelvis (50%): normal female type, inlet is slightly transverse and oval; the sacrum is wide with average concavity and inclination; the subpubic angle is 90–100°.
- Anthropoid pelvis (25%): ape-like; anteroposterior (AP) diameters are long; transverse diameter is short; the sacrum is long and narrow, the subpubic angle is narrow.
- Android pelvis (20%): male type, the pelvic inlet is triangular or heart-shaped with an anterior narrow apex, subpubic angle is narrow < 90°.
- Platypelloid pelvis (5%): flat female type, AP diameter is short, transverse diameter is long and subpubic angle is wide.

7. D Pubococcygeus

The levator ani muscle is formed by the pubococcygeus, iliococcygeus and ischiococcygeus. Although considered in three parts, the muscle forms a continuous sheet, which provides significant support to the pelvic organs. Pubococcygeus forms the bulk of the levator ani muscle, arising from the back of the pubis and the white line that runs in front of the obturator canal. Its fibres form a U-shaped loop, which runs around the urethra, vagina and anorectal junction, with the medial fibres blending with the upper urethra. Intermediate fibres loop around the vagina, closing the lower end on contraction. Lateral fibres run around the anus, inserting into the lateral and posterior walls of the anal canal between the internal and external sphincters. Iliococcygeus arises from the white line behind the obturator canal and inserts into the lateral margins of the coccyx. Ischiococcygeus arises from ischial spine and inserts into the coccyx.

8. A Adrenal gland inner medulla

The adrenal glands are retroperitoneal endocrine organs situated near the kidneys. They are surrounded by adipose tissue and renal fascia and are usually found at the level of the 12th thoracic vertebra. The outer cortex is mainly responsible for the synthesis of corticosteroid hormones and aldosterone and is derived from coelomic mesothelium. The inner medulla chromaffin cells are the source of catecholamines and these cells are derived from ectodermal neural crest cells.

9. B Anterior division L2–L4

The obturator nerve arises from the anterior division of L2–L4. It emerges from the medial border of the psoas major and descends along the muscle. It runs above and in front of the obturator vessels. It passes through the obturator foramen and enters the thigh through the obturator canal. After passing through the obturator canal, it divides into an anterior and a posterior branch. The anterior branch provides an articular branch to the hip and anterior adductor muscles. The obturator nerve provides sensory innervation to the skin on the medial surface of the thigh. The posterior branch innervates the deeper adductor muscles. The femoral nerve is formed from the posterior division of L2–L4.

10. B Facilitated diffusion

As there is normally no mixing of fetal and maternal blood, a selective transport of different nutrients and waste products across the placenta is required. Gases such as oxygen and carbon dioxide are able to use simple diffusion to cross the placenta in response to gradients in partial pressures. The partial pressure of carbon dioxide is greater in fetal blood and thus is diffused into the maternal circulation to be expired from the maternal lungs. The partial pressure of oxygen is greater in the maternal circulation, thus diffuses into the fetal blood.

Glucose is the main energy source for the fetus; it is transported across the placenta by facilitated diffusion via GLUT 3 and GLUT 1 transporters. Amino acid is transported by active transport from the maternal blood, as the concentrations are higher than in the fetal blood.

11. D Placenta

Alkaline phosphatase (ALP) increases throughout normal pregnancy due to the production of the placenta, and can reach three times the normal adult upper reference value. Albumin levels often decrease in pregnancy due to haemodilution, as do the levels of the transaminases and gamma-glutamyltransferase (GGT). Therefore, elevated levels of alanine transaminase (ALT) are not normal and should be investigated.

Below is a table of the normal values for pregnancy of the liver function tests.

Table 15.2 Normal values for liver function tests

Liver function tests	Pre-pregnancy levels	3rd trimester pregnancy levels
ALT (IU/L)	0–40	6–32
Aspartate transaminase (IU/L)	7–40	11–30
Bilirubin (µmol/L)	0–17	3–14
GGT (IU/L)	11–50	3–41
ALP (IU/L)	30–130	133–418
Albumin (g/L)	35–46	28–37
Bile acids (µmol/L)	0–14	0–14

Adapted from Walker I, Chappell C, Williamson C. Abnormal liver function tests in pregnancy. BMJ 2013; 347:f6055 doi: 10.1136/bmj.f6055

12. B Gestational diabetes

Testing for gestational diabetes should be performed with a 2-hour 75 g oral glucose tolerance test (OGTT) in women with one or more risk factors at 24–28 weeks' gestation. Risk factors include body mass index above 30 kg/m², previous gestational diabetes, previous macrosomic baby weighing 4.5 kg or above, minority ethnic family origin with high prevalence of diabetes, or positive family history of diabetes.

Gestational diabetes is diagnosed if either:

- A fasting plasma glucose level of 5.6 mmol/litre or above, or
- A 2-hour plasma glucose level of 7.8 mmol/litre or above.

13. E Metanephros – kidney

Gonadal development begins at the mesonephros during the fourth week. The clitoris is formed from the genital tubercle. Initially the gonads are swellings and there is no differentiation until the seventh week. The SRY gene determines sex differentiation, and is located on the short arm of chromosome 11. In the female embryo the gonads develop from the paramesonephric ducts. The genital folds form the labia minora and the genital swellings the labia majora. The bladder and urethra are derived from the primitive urogenital sinus and the ureters from the ureteric bud. Three excretory systems develop: pronephros, mesonephros and finally the metanephros, from which the kidney is developed.

14. D The cardinal vein runs into the sinus venosus

There are two umbilical arteries and one vein. The ligamentum venosum is a remnant of the ductus venosus and is found on the inferior surface of the liver.

The ductus venosus is a variation of the fetal circulation, which directs blood from the umbilical vein into the inferior vena cava. This allows oxygenated blood from the placenta to bypass the liver. The cardiac system is developed from angiogenic mesoderm cells. The anterior cardinal vein forms the internal jugular vein and combined with the common cardinal vein forms the superior vena cava. The cardinal vein drains into the sinus venosus.

15. B Inferior mesenteric vein

The vitelline veins bring blood away from the yolk sac. The vitelline veins give rise to the hepatic veins, the inferior part of the inferior vena cava, the superior mesenteric vein and the portal vein. The inferior mesenteric vein is not a derivative of the vitelline vein.

16. A Sex cords are developed from coelomic epithelium

Sex differentiation occurs in the ninth week after fertilisation. Reproductive organs develop from intermediate mesoderm, rather than paraxial mesoderm. The gubernaculum assists in the descent of the gonads in both sexes. In males only the lower part persists to become the scrotal ligament. In females, the upper part becomes the ovarian ligament and the lower part becomes the round ligament of the uterus.

17. D Hypotension, hyperkalaemia and hyponatraemia

90% of patients with congenital adrenal hyperplasia (CAH) have 21-hydroxylase deficiency. This enzyme has a function in both the production of glucocorticoids and mineralocorticoids, and therefore patients may have a 'salt-wasting' syndrome. A deficiency in mineralocorticoids leads to hypotension as a result of hypovolaemia, with hyponatraemia and hyperkalaemia. See **Figure 15.2** for steroidogenesis pathways.

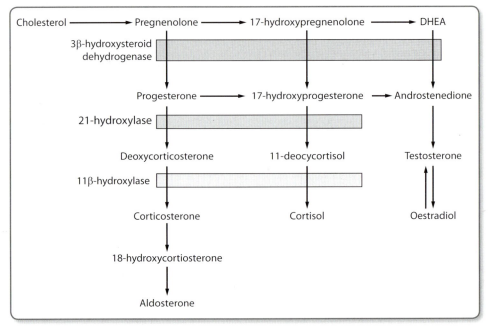

Figure 15.2 Steroidogenesis pathways.

10% of patients with CAH have a deficiency of 11β-hydroxylase. In this instance there remains a deficiency of glucocorticoids; however, there is an accumulation of deoxycortisol, which may cause hypertension due to its glucocorticoid properties.

18. E Reduced plasma iodine concentration in early pregnancy

During the first trimester, the increased renal blood flow and glomerular filtration rate lead to increased level of iodine clearance from the plasma. Patients with already low levels of iodine are predisposed to developing goitre. In the first trimester, rising levels of human chorionic gonadotrophin (hCG) lead to a reduction in serum levels of thyroid-stimulating hormone (TSH) as it has thyrotropic properties, because of the structural similarity of hCG to TSH. Pregnancy is associated with increased thyroid binding globulin because of increased liver production, with subsequent elevation of total T4 and T3.

19. A It enhances amino acid transfer across the placenta

Human placental lactogen (HPL) is one of several peptides made by the placenta. Its structure and function is similar to growth hormone. It affects the maternal metabolism to provide increased nutrient supply to the fetus. HPL decreases maternal insulin sensitivity and therefore leads to greater amount of glucose in the blood. Lipolysis is induced which leads to fatty acids being released into the bloodstream. HPL decreases maternal glucose utilisation. HPL is only present in pregnancy and reaches its highest concentration by the third trimester. It has previously been used as an indicator of fetal wellbeing.

20. A Conversion of cholesterol to pregnenolone

All steroids are synthesised from cholesterol, with the first step of the pathway being the conversion of cholesterol to pregnenolone by cholesterol monooxygenase. Dihydrotesterone is produced from oestradiol by 5-alpha reductase (See **Figure 15.2**).

21. E Increase gluconeogenesis

The action of cortisol can be summarised as follows:

- Increasing plasma glucose
- Increase gluconeogenesis
- Increase glycogenesis
- Increase glycogen storage
- Increase lipolysis
- Increase protein catabolism
- Sodium and water retention
- Anti-inflammatory
- Increased gastric acid production

22. A Diabetes insipidus

Cushing's syndrome is a state of excess of cortisol. Characteristic features include: truncal obesity, a red puffy rounded face, hypertension, depression, osteoporosis, diabetes mellitus, striae, hirsuitism and amenorrhoea. Causes of excess cortisol production fall into four main categories:

1. Latrogenic
2. Excess adrenocorticotrophic hormone (ACTH) production by pituitary tumour (Cushing's disease)
3. Adrenal cortical neoplasm producing steroid
4. Ectopic production of ACTH by non-pituitary tumour (e.g. lung tumour)

23. C Low-dose dexamethasone suppression test

The best screening test is the overnight dexamethasone suppression test, which is used to eliminate all those with no abnormality. False positives will be seen in alcoholics, those with anorexia nervosa and anyone taking enzyme inducer medication. If this test is positive, then further tests are done to localise the disease.

Low-dose dexamethasone suppression test involves giving 0.5 mg/6 hours orally for 48 hours and then measuring plasma cortisol at 0 hours and 48 hours. This test is used to confirm the diagnosis. Localisation of the disease is subsequently delineated via the high dose dexamethasone test (complete or partial suppression indicates Cushing's disease) and testing plasma adrenocorticotrophic hormone level.

24. C Hypokalaemia

Cushing's syndrome is a disorder of high serum cortisol, which has many causes and has been discussed previously. The most common cause is exogenous administration of steroid hormones. Cushing's disease refers to Cushing's syndrome caused specifically by a tumour of the pituitary gland, which secretes large amounts of adrenocorticotropic hormone, leading to high cortisol. Patients may have hyperglycaemia and insulin resistance, causing diabetes mellitus. Findings of hyperglycaemia and hypokalaemia may be accompanied by hypernatraemia as a result of increased aldosterone levels. It may also lead to metabolic alkalosis.

25. C 4

The standard deviation of a sample is a measure of the scatter of the data set around the mean. The variance is a measure of how far each observation within the sample varies from the mean. Knowledge of the basic formula used to calculate standard deviation is key to answering this question. The standard deviation can be calculated by taking the square root of the variance. There are other formulas that can be used to calculate the standard deviation but from the limited information given this simple formula should be used.

Worked answer:

Standard deviation = square root of the variance

Variance = 16

Square root of 16 = 4

Therefore, the standard deviation = 4

26. B To assess the extent to which current practice meets a defined set of standards

It is important to be able to distinguish the difference between research and audit. Both are integral to the advancement of medical knowledge and clinical practice.

Of the statements given for this question, only the stem 'to assess the extent to which current practice meets a defined set of standards' is a valid aim of audit. The other stems actually refer to aims of research studies. Audit should occur regularly within a clinical setting to assess how practice standards are being met and the need to implement strategies for improvement. The process of audit is described as a continuous cycle, starting with defining the standards of the area of interest, collecting data, making an assessment of current practice and whether it meets the standards, followed by identifying and implementing any required changes in practice.

27. D 8

Calculating relative risk is a means of quantifying the risk of an event, or a disease relative to exposure to a contributory factor. A calculated relative risk of an event/ condition equal to 1 indicates that there is no difference between those who were exposed to the factor and those who were not. A relative risk of less than one suggests that the exposure group is less likely to develop the condition than the non-exposure group, whereas a relative risk greater than one indicates that the risk of condition is increased in the exposure group relative to the non-exposure group. For this study, the calculated relative risk of women with gestational diabetes mellitus (GDM), in this study, delivering a baby weighing > 4.5 kg was eight. This indicates that women with GDM had eight times the risk of having a baby weighing > 4.5 kg. **Table 15.3** sets out the groups for calculation of relative risk.

Table 15.3 Calculating relative risk

Event/condition of interest	Exposed group	Non-exposed group	Total
Yes	A	B	A + B
No	C	D	C + D
Total	A + C	B + D	A + B + C + D

Relative risk can be calculated as below:

Relative risk $= \dfrac{A/(A + C)}{B/(B + D)}$

Using the data supplied in the question:

Proportion of diabetic mothers with babies > 4.5 kg $= 80/200 = 0.4$

Proportion of non-diabetic mothers with babies > 4.5 kg $= 50/1000 = 0.05$

Relative risk of diabetic women delivering a baby weighing 4.5 kg $= 0.4/0.05 = 8$

Relative risk $= \dfrac{80/(80 + 120)}{50/(50 + 950)} = 8$

28. B 2a

Research can be given a level of the evidence, and further graded A–C using the below accepted hierarchy.

Level	Type of evidence source	Grade
I	Randomised controlled trial (RCT) or a meta-analysis of RCTs	A
II a	At least one well-designed un-randomised study	B
II b	At least one well-designed experimental study	
III	A well-designed non-experimental descriptive studies (e.g. comparative studies, case studies)	
IV	Expert committee reports or opinions and/or clinical experiences of respected authorities	C

29. A Each consists of two identical chromatids

Chromosomes consist of long strands of DNA, which have been elaborately folded and coiled. Within the strands of DNA are sequences, which are genes. In eukaryotic cells, they are found in the cell nuclei, where the DNA material is packaged as chromatin. Each chromosome consists of two identical chromatids, which are held together in the midline at the centromere. The shape of chromosomes may be described according to the position of the centromere. The short arm of a chromosome is known as the p arm, whereas the long arm is known as the q arm. Humans have 22 autosomal chromosome pairs and one pair of sex chromosomes

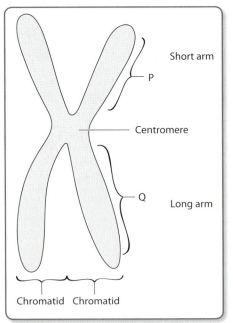

Figure 15.3 Basic structure of a chromosome.

in each cell. Chromosomes are best visualised in the metaphase of mitosis. Giemsa staining may be used to aid visualisation of gene rich areas, which aids chromosome identification in a process called G-banding. See **Figure 15.3** for the basic structure of a chromosome.

30. E It is caused by a defect in the cystic fibrosis transmembrane conductance gene

Cystic fibrosis (CF) is an autosomal recessive condition affecting exocrine function. CF is typically found in Caucasian populations and is considered a life-limiting condition. It is often associated with manifestations such as severe lung disease, pancreatic insufficiency and infertility. CF is caused by a defect in the CF transmembrane conductance regulator (CFTR) gene found on chromosome 7. This leads to a defect in the CTFR protein, which acts as a chloride channel. Defective transport of chloride ions across epithelial cell membranes and an accumulation of intracellular sodium causes an excess of thick secretions on mucosal surfaces. CF is caused by a large number of mutations in the CFTR gene; however, the most commonly identified defect is a deletion of the 508th codon of the gene, leading to the absence of a phenylalanine residue. This mutation is usually denoted as ΔF508.

31. B Cri-du-chat

A series of syndromes have been identified that arise due to chromosomal microdeletions. A microdeletion refers to the loss of a small subset of genes, which are found adjacent to each other on a chromosome. Syndromes caused by microdeletions tend to have common characteristics including learning difficulties, dysmorphic facial features and organ abnormalities such as cardiac anomalies. Many cases of Angelman syndrome are caused by a microdeletion associated with the loss the maternally inherited chromosome 15; its equivalent is Prader–Willi syndrome, which can be caused by loss of the paternally inherited chromosome 15. Di-George and Shprintzen-Goldberg syndromes are both associated with deletion of the proximal long arm of chromosome 22. Cri-du-chat syndrome is caused by a loss of part of the short arm of chromosome 5 (**Table 15.4**).

Table 15.4 Examples of syndromes caused by chromosome microdeletions

Microdeletion syndrome	Chromosome affected
Cri-du-chat	5
Williams	7
Angelman	15
Prader–Willi	15
Smith–Magenis	17
Di-George	22

32. A Trisomy 16 is the most common trisomy in miscarried fetuses

Aneuploidy refers to an abnormal number of chromosomes and can occur both to autosomes and the sex chromosomes. The majority of trisomies occur following a non-disjunction event, which occurs in the meiotic division. The most common trisomy found in miscarried fetuses is trisomy 16, which is incompatible with life. Trisomy 21 is the most common trisomy compatible with life. Babies with trisomies 13 and 18 have a considerably shortened life expectancy, with the majority not surviving infancy. Individuals with a trisomy of the X chromosome typically have normal lives and their aneuploidy is often not diagnosed. The loss of an autosome, i.e. a monosomy of a chromosome, is not compatible with life; however, fetuses affected by the monosomy of the X sex chromosome, i.e. Turner's syndrome, can survive (albeit with a high incidence of miscarriage). Noonan's syndrome is an autosomal recessive condition associated with mutations of four genes leading to multiple organ defects.

33. D Metaplasia

Cervical ectropion is a normal occurrence caused by hyper-oestrogenic states such as the ovulatory phase in younger women, pregnancy and use of the oral contraceptive pill. The endocervical columnar epithelium protrudes out of the external os, before undergoing squamous metaplasia. It transforms into stratified squamous epithelium. It may lead to increased vaginal discharge and contact (e.g. post-coital) bleeding.

34. C Low FSH:LH ratio, low SHBG

Polycystic ovarian syndrome (PCOS) can be diagnosed using the Rotterdam consensus (2003) criteria. This states that the patient must fulfil two of the following three criteria.

1. Clinical or biochemical hyperandrogenism
2. Oligomenorrhea or oligo-ovulation
3. Polycystic ovaries on ultrasound ($\geq$ 12 antral follicles in one ovary or ovarian volume $\geq$ 10 cm^3)

Not included in the diagnostic criteria but characteristic to PCOS are the biochemical changes which include:

- FSH levels are either normal or low, LH levels are elevated, and the LH-FSH ratio is usually greater than 3
- Levels of sex hormone binding globulin (SHBG) are usually low
- There is a high prevalence of impaired glucose tolerance and type 2 diabetes in women with PCOS

35. A High SHBG, high oestradiol, high progesterone

Sex hormone binding globulin (SHBG) is a glycoprotein that binds to the sex hormones testosterone and oestrogen. Only a small amount of circulating testosterone and oestrogen is 'free', with most bound to SHBG. The liver produces most SHBG. SHBG levels increase with hyper-estrogenic states such as pregnancy or combined oral contraceptive pill use.

Progesterone levels increase throughout pregnancy. They are produced by the corpus luteum until implantation of the embryo, after which the placenta is the site of production.

The three main types of oestrogen are oestrone, oestradiol and oestriol. Oestradiol is the principal oestrogen during the reproductive years. Oestriol is the predominant oestrogen circulating during pregnancy. Oestrone is the predominant oestrogen during the menopause

Cortisol is a glucocorticoid hormone produced by the adrenal cortex (in the zona fasciculata), which modulates the response to stress. During pregnancy, increased fetal cortisol occurs during weeks 30–32 and triggers production of surfactant.

36. E Proximal tubule

The proximal tubule is responsible for reabsorption of approximately two thirds of the urine volume and electrolytes. Water reabsorption is a passive process of osmosis, driven by the gradient of electrolyte concentrations.

Approximately 90% of the bicarbonate filtered through the glomerulus is reabsorbed within the proximal tubule, the remainder occurring in the ascending loop of Henle and the collecting duct. The filtered bicarbonate ions and the secreted hydrogen ions form carbonic anhydrase, which dissociates to form water and carbon dioxide molecules. These carbon dioxide molecules enter into the tubule cell and bind with hydroxide ion to form bicarbonate. In normal pH states, the bicarbonate is reabsorbed through the sodium/bicarbonate co-transporter, and in cases of alkalosis the bicarbonate can be secreted.

37. E 99%

The vast majority of calcium is stored in the skeleton (99%), with less than 1% stored intracellularly and only 0.1% extracellularly. Of the extracellular component, 45% is ionised and thus physiological, whereas 55% is bound to mainly plasma proteins and to lesser extent anions. Calcium requirements increase from 1 g to 1.5 g daily during pregnancy and lactation.

38. B Absorption of fats

Obstetric cholestasis in pregnancy is characterised by pruritus (classically affecting the soles and palms) in the absence of skin rash with abnormal liver function tests and/or raised bile acids, neither of which has an alternative cause and both of which resolve after birth. In pregnancies complicated by obstetric cholestasis, there is an increased risk to the fetus, including preterm birth and stillbirth.

No treatment has been shown to improve fetal outcomes. Ursodeoxycholic acid can improve pruritus and liver function tests. Vitamin K should be considered if the prothrombin time is prolonged.

39. C Pressure on the inferior vena cava

Many physiological changes occur during pregnancy. It is important to have a clear understanding of these to avoid mis-interpreting these changes as pathological; the table below summarises the cardiovascular and haematological changes seen in pregnancy. In this scenario, the patient has worsening varicose veins, and in pregnancy the most likely cause is mechanical compression on the inferior vena cava by the gravid uterus. Other features including hormonal changes causing vasodilation, and increased plasma volume are also likely to contribute.

Table 15.5 Cardiovascular and haematological physiological changes in pregnancy	
Plasma volume	Increases to 2600-3800 mL (by 6-8 weeks; no increase after 32 weeks)
Red cell mass	Increases to 1400-1800 mL (steady increase until term)
Cardiac output	Increases to 4.5-6.0 L/min (early in pregnancy; no increase after 24-30 weeks)
	Distribution to uterus and skin increases in third trimester; increases to kidneys and breasts early in pregnancy
Stroke volume	Increases early in pregnancy
Heart rate	Increases late in pregnancy to 80-90 bpm
Blood pressure	Peripheral vascular resistance reduces; systolic decrease by 5 mmHg; diastolic decrease by 10 mmHg
ECG changes	Left ventricular hypertrophy leads to left axis deviation. Heart rate increases
	Displacement of diaphragm upwards leads to apex being shifted anterior and left
	Inverted T waves in I Lead III / Q wave Lead III and avF / ST changes non-specific

40. D Increases by 30–40%

Physiological changes to the respiratory system in pregnancy

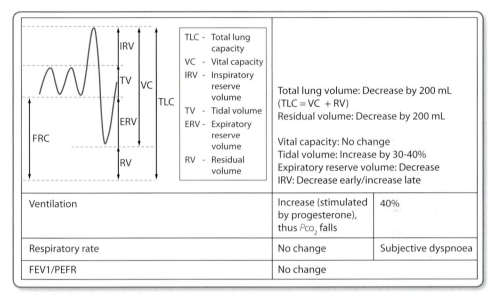

	Total lung volume: Decrease by 200 mL (TLC = VC + RV) Residual volume: Decrease by 200 mL Vital capacity: No change Tidal volume: Increase by 30-40% Expiratory reserve volume: Decrease IRV: Decrease early/increase late	
Ventilation	Increase (stimulated by progesterone), thus P_{CO_2} falls	40%
Respiratory rate	No change	Subjective dyspnoea
FEV1/PEFR	No change	

Figure 15.4 Physiological changes in pregnancy.

41. C Pyramidalis

Pyramidalis is a triangular muscle, which lies within the rectus sheath in front of the rectus abdominis. It is absent in 20% of people and is supplied by the subcostal nerve. The subcostal nerve is the anterior branch of the 12th thoracic nerve. It communicates with the iliohypogastric nerve and gives a branch to pyramidalis. It gives off a lateral cutaneous nerve supplying sensory innervation to the skin over the hip.

42. B Iliacus

Iliacus is separated from extraperitoneal tissue by the iliac fascia. It has a wide peripheral attachment to the iliac crest, which it shares with the psoas muscle and descends to leave the abdomen behind the inguinal ligament. The iliacus muscle has innervation from the femoral nerve and lumbar plexus. The iliacus and psoas muscles act in synergy to flex the hip joint.

43. A External oblique

The external oblique arises from the outer surface and lower borders of the eight lowest ribs, passing downwards and backwards. The aponeurosis forms part of the inguinal ligament. See **Figure 15.5** for the anatomy of the inguinal canal.

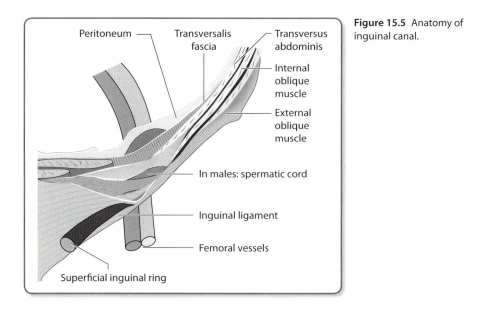

Figure 15.5 Anatomy of inguinal canal.

Labels in figure:
Peritoneum — Transversalis fascia — Transversus abdominis — Internal oblique muscle — External oblique muscle — In males: spermatic cord — Inguinal ligament — Femoral vessels — Superficial inguinal ring

44. D Superior epigastric artery

The superior epigastric artery is a terminal branch of the internal thoracic artery and forms an anastomosis with the inferior epigastric artery. It pierces the rectus sheath and anastomoses with the inferior epigastric artery at the level of the umbilicus. It supplies the anterior part of the abdominal wall and some of the diaphragm. It has a corresponding vein, the superior epigastric vein.

45. C Superior gluteal artery

The superior gluteal artery is one of three branches of the posterior division of the internal iliac artery, the other two being the iliolumbar and the lateral sacral arteries. The superior vesical artery continues as the obliterated umbilical artery after supplying the lower ureter and upper bladder. The uterine artery runs medially on levator ani, in front of the ureter and above the lateral vaginal fornix. Once it has supplied the ureteric and vaginal branches it ascends the side of the uterus to anastomose with the ovarian artery.

46. E L2 and L3

The lateral cutaneous nerve of the thigh is a cutaneous nerve originating from the lumbar plexus. It arises from the dorsal division of L2 and L3. It emerges laterally on the psoas muscle and after crossing the iliacus muscle, passes under the inguinal ligament and divides into anterior and posterior branches.

47. C Pelvic splanchnic nerves

Pelvic splanchnic nerves are autonomic nerves that arise from the ventral rami of S2–S4, providing parasympathetic innervation. This parasympathetic outflow supplies part of the gut, bladder, genitals and blood vessels in the pelvis, releasing acetylcholine at its terminals. They also carry visceral afferent fibres. The pelvic splanchnic nerves communicate with the inferior hypogastric plexus located at each side of the rectum and vagina. From here the nerves are distributed locally and up through the inferior hypogastric nerve and superior hypogastric plexus. Afferent fibres from the cervix travel within the pelvic splanchnic nerves to the dorsal roots of the upper sacral nerves.

48. A Columnar epithelium

The uterus is lined by endometrium. The endometrium consists of a single layer of columnar epithelial cells, which rest on a layer of connective tissue (stroma). Secretory glands and spiral arteries extend from the surface of the endometrium to the base of the stroma.

49. D Stratified squamous epithelium

The urethra originates from endoderm and arises from the pelvic part of the urogenital sinus. The proximal half of the urethra is lined with transitional epithelium and the distal half is lined with stratified squamous epithelium.

50. D Round ligament

The uterosacral ligaments extend from the posterior cervix to the sacrum. As they pull the cervix backwards, they help hold the uterus in an anteverted position, as well as providing support for the uterus and vagina. The round ligament is approximately 12 cm long and runs from the body of the uterus in front of and below the insertion of the fallopian tube to the internal inguinal ring. It traverses the inguinal canal and exits from the external inguinal ring, breaking up into strands at the labium majus. In the fetus a peritoneal tube, the processus vaginalis, surrounds the round ligament. This is usually obliterated at birth, however, it occasionally persists and if this is the case it can be a site for hernia development. The broad ligament is a double fold of peritoneum, providing no role in the support of the uterus.

51. D Middle rectal artery

Contents of the ischiorectal fossa include:

- Inferior rectal nerve and vessels
- Pudendal canal and its contents
- Fat pad
- Perforating cutaneous branch of S2 and S3
- Perineal branch of S4
- Labial nerve and vein

52. A Above pectinate line: derived endoderm, superior rectal artery

The pectinate line lies at the junction of the upper two-thirds and the lower one-third of the anal canal. Embryologically this represents the junction of the hindgut and the proctodeum (**Table 15.5**).

Table 15.5 Anatomy and embryology of the anal canal		
	Above pectinate line	**Below pectinate line**
Epithelium	Columnar	Stratified squamous
Embryological origin	Endoderm	Ectoderm
Artery	Superior rectal artery	Middle and inferior rectal artery
Vein	Superior rectal vein	Middle and inferior rectal vein
Nerves	Inferior hypogastric plexus	Inferior rectal nerves

53. A Lateral wall of ischiorectal fossa; above sacrotuberous ligament

The pudendal canal is a tunnel of fascia that runs in the lower lateral wall of the ischiorectal fossa, just above the sacrotuberous ligament. It contains the pudendal nerve and the internal pudendal vessels. During a pudendal block, the pudendal nerve is infiltrated where it crosses the ischial spine. It is reached through the vagina and infiltrated medial to the ischial spine.

54. D Stratified squamous

The female urethra is lined by transitional epithelium proximal to the bladder and by stratified squamous epithelium in its distal portion. It is endodermal in origin from the urogenital sinus. It takes its blood supply from the inferior vesical artery and the internal pudendal artery with drainage to the vesical plexus. Lymphatic drainage is to the internal iliac lymph nodes.

55. B T7–T12

The rectus abdominis muscle originates at the pubis muscle and has its insertion into the costal cartilages of the fifth, sixth and seventh ribs and the sternum. It is contained within the rectus sheath, which is made up of the aponeuroses of the external and internal oblique muscle and the transversus abdominis muscle. The external oblique is the most superficial aponeurosis to make up the rectus sheath and has the internal oblique beneath it to keep it separate from the rectus muscle. It is supplied by the inferior epigastric artery and has its nerve supply from the thoracoabdominal nerves, T7–T12.

56. D Rickets

This 4-year-old boy is suffering from rickets, which is caused by failure or delay to mineralise endochondral bone in the growth plate. The main cause is impaired metabolism or deficiency of vitamin D. His mother is complaining of premenstrual symptoms, combined with bony pain. These are symptoms of vitamin D deficiency in adults. Treatment for both of these patients would be to ensure adequate sunlight exposure and prescribe vitamin D supplements. Vitamin D is required for adequate absorption of calcium and is synthesised in the skin following sunlight exposure and from the kidney.

Osteopetrosis, also known as marble bone disease, is caused by a deficiency of osteoclasts. There is hardening of the bones and an elevation in levels of alkaline phosphatase. Perthes' disease is a disease of the hip joint, caused by avascular necrosis of the femoral head and a reduction in blood supply. Scurvy is caused by a lack of vitamin C and symptoms may include gum disease, easy bruising and myalgia.

57. C Multiple myeloma

Multiple myeloma is a neoplastic expansion of plasma cells within the blood, with an incidence of 5/100,000. Proliferation of plasma cells interferes with normal production of blood cells within the bone marrow, resulting in anaemia, leucopenia and thrombocytopaenia. Presentation of this condition includes bone pain, pathological fractures and renal failure. Diagnosis is via electrophoresis of serum and/or urine, identifying a monoclonal paraprotein. Bence Jones proteins (immunoglobulin light chains) may be identified in the urine. Patients develop hypercalcaemia due to excessive tumour-induced osteoclast-mediated bone destruction, caused by cytokines expressed or secreted locally at myeloma cells. This leads to an efflux of calcium into extracellular fluid. Treatment is supportive, with correction of renal failure and hypercalcaemia.

58. B Hyperglycaemia

A glucagonoma is a tumour of the α cells of the pancreas. It is associated with excessive production of glucagon. Glucagon can be thought of as acting in opposition to insulin, therefore raising serum glucose levels through gluconeogenesis and lipolysis. This rare tumour is characterised by a state of extreme hyperglycaemia due to excessive levels of glucagon. Other manifestations include a characteristic rash and anaemia. Although incredibly rare, this tumour is more common in perimenopausal and postmenopausal women.

59. D pH 7.50, P_{CO_2} 3.0 kPa, P_{O_2} 9.2 kPa, HCO_3 25.0 mmol/L

This patient has an acute pulmonary embolus (PE). PE is a relatively common postoperative complication and clinical presentation includes chest pain, dyspnoea and haemoptysis. Signs and symptoms in this case are the acute dyspnoea and pain on inspiration. The low oxygen saturations and tachycardia would also be found in patients with acute PE. It usually occurs when thrombosis from a more distal vein breaks loose and embolises into pulmonary blood vessels. The arterial blood gas in a patient with a PE most commonly shows respiratory alkalosis. The low partial pressure of carbon dioxide is most likely caused by hyperventilation. In cases of massive PE, the infarcted or non-functioning areas of the lung may lead to increased P_{CO_2} values. Hypoxaemia occurs due to altered areas of perfusion and ventilation of the lung tissue (VQ mismatch). Although a pH of 7.2 is reasonable, this patient is extremely unlikely to have a P_{O_2} of 12.0 kPa, given oxygen saturation of 93%.

60. A pH 7.16, P_{CO_2} 8.2 kPa, P_{O_2} 15.3 kPa, HCO_3 21.2 mmol/L

This patient has central respiratory depression due to opiate overdose. Fatty liver of pregnancy may be associated with an acid–base abnormality if it is severe. Symptoms include fatigue, nausea and vomiting, and upper abdominal pain, usually in the third trimester. The pattern on arterial blood gas usually shows a mixed metabolic and respiratory acidosis, reflected in the degree of acidosis.

The Henderson–Hasselbach equation describes the relationship of pH as a measure of acidity.

pH = pKa + log

Where pKa is the acid dissociation constant.

61. A High blood levels of fatty acids

There are profound changes in the metabolism of fat during episodes of diabetic ketoacidosis. There are high blood levels of fatty acids and lactate. Blood pH may drop to below 7.0 and the kidney excretes hydrogen ions to compensate. The state of metabolic acidosis causes an activation of chemoreceptors in the brain, which subsequently leads to hyperventilation. Patients are usually severely dehydrated due to a state of osmotic diuresis and hyperglycaemia, and often hypoxic. Diabetic ketoacidosis is a medical emergency and should be treated promptly. Treatment involves controlled replacement of fluids, including correction of electrolyte imbalance. A sliding scale should also be in place until normal glucose control can be initiated.

62. A Prostacyclin PGI2

All of the options given are prostaglandins, thromboxanes or prostacyclins. Classified together as prostanoids, which are forms of eicosanoids. These fatty acid derivatives are all formed from the conversion of arachidonic acid via the action of cyclooxygenase (COX). Prostacyclin PGI2 is formed from the conversion of arachidonic acid to prostaglandin H2, which is then converted to its final form by the action of prostacyclin synthase. Released by endothelial cells, prostacyclin

PGI2 acts predominantly to inhibit platelet aggregation via activation of G-protein coupled receptors on the platelet surface, leading to production of cyclic adenosine monophosphate with subsequent inhibition of platelet activation. Prostcyclin PGI2 also acts as a vasodilator. Thromboxane TXA2 is a prothrombotic, which is produced by activated platelets, which acts to promote platelet activation and vasoconstriction.

63. B Ampulla of the fallopian tube

The ovum is carried from the ovary into the fallopian tube following ovulation. It is picked up by the fimbriae and carried into the tube. Inside the fallopian tube the ovum is moved medially by the action of cilia lining the tube and muscular action. The ovum is halted at the fallopian ampulla for up to 36 hours and therefore fertilisation occurs at this location most frequently.

64. B Vitellointestinal duct

Meckel's diverticulum is an abnormality of the midgut. It occurs in 2–4% of the population and is a common anomaly of the digestive system. It is more common in males than females and is a persistence of the vitellointestinal duct. The vitellointestinal duct is present in early embryonic life and its function is to provide nutrition to the yolk sac. It usually regresses by the seventh week. A Meckel diverticulum is a blind ending tube and contains all the layers of gut that are present in the ileum. It is located approximately 50–60 cm from the ileocaecal valve. If this remnant becomes inflamed, it may produce a condition with a similar presentation to appendicitis. The mucosa is gastric in origin and may therefore produce gastric acid, which may lead to ulceration and bleeding.

65. D Prostate

The mesonephric duct ultimately gives rise to several parts of the male urogenital tract, including the epididymis, the vas deferens and the seminal vesicle. The prostate is not derived from the mesonephric duct and develops from the urogenital sinus.

66. D Shortened Q–T interval and widened T wave on ECG

Hypercalcaemia may cause ECG changes, specifically a shortened QT interval and a widened T wave complex. Hypocalcaemia may lead to many classic signs and symptoms, one of which is a prolonged Q–T interval on ECG. Circumoral tingling and numbness, carpopedal spasm and depression are all symptoms of hypocalcaemia. Chvostek's sign may be positive, twitching of the face with tapping of the facial nerve. Trousseau's sign is a carpopedal spasm, which can be induced by inflating a blood pressure cuff around the arm. Calcium levels may be misinterpreted if the albumin levels are abnormal and therefore calculation should always take this into account.

67. D 21α-hydroxylase

Congenital adrenal hyperplasia (CAH) is an autosomal recessive disorder, which occurs as a result of a defect in the pathway of steroidogenesis in the adrenal gland. As a result of this, there is cortisol deficiency and increased androgen production. The majority of cases occur as a result in deficiency of the enzyme 21α-hydroxylase. CAH is rare and occurs in approximately 1 in 14,000 births. Presentation of this syndrome may include salt wasting if production of aldosterone is affected and hypoglycaemia may occur. Neonates may have ambiguous genitalia and, despite a 46 XX genotype, may appear male. Diagnosis is made via detection of 17-hydroxyprogesterone levels. It may also be necessary to perform a 24-hour urinary steroid analysis.

68. D Phenytoin

Hirsutism is the presence of hair on the body and face that grows in excess. It is usually in a male pattern of growth and is caused by an excess of testosterone. It is associated with polycystic ovarian syndrome and alopecia.

The Ferriman–Gallwey score may be used to grade hirsutism and uses a score of 0–4 ranging from no hair cover (0) to fully hair covered (4) in 9 areas of the body: upper lip, chest, chin, upper abdomen, lower abdomen, upper and lower back, upper arms and thighs. A score above 8 suggests possible androgen excess.

Other drug causes include danazol, progesterones (including the combined oral contraceptive pill), metoclopramide, methyldopa, anabolic steroids, reserpine, testosterone, cyclosporine, minoxidil and diazoxide.

69. B Basophils of the anterior pituitary gland

Thyroid-stimulating hormone (TSH) is produced by the basophils of anterior pituitary gland. High levels of T4 and T3 lead to a reduction in the production of both TSH and thyrotrophin-releasing hormone (TRH) via the feedback loop, as shown in **Figure 15.6**. The same mechanism means that high levels of TSH lead to a reduction in production of TRH. TRH is produced by the paraventricular nucleus of the hypothalamus.

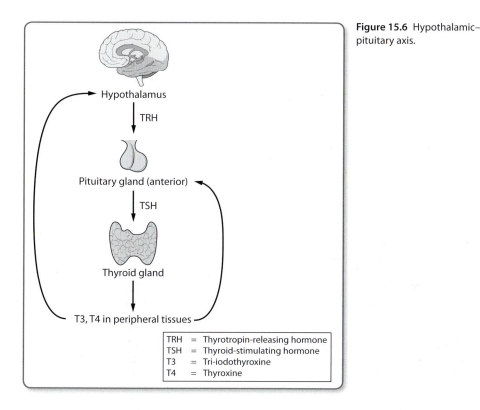

Figure 15.6 Hypothalamic–pituitary axis.

TRH	=	Thyrotropin-releasing hormone
TSH	=	Thyroid-stimulating hormone
T3	=	Tri-iodothyroxine
T4	=	Thyroxine

70. E All of the above

Hyperthyroidism produces a range of symptoms that occur as a result of increased production of thyroid hormones. Symptoms include diarrhoea, weight loss, increased appetite, psychosis, heat intolerance, oligomenorrhoea and infertility. In many circumstances, infertility may be how the disease is detected.

71. B Bicarbonate

Calcium is essential for the regulation of the nervous and musculoskeletal systems, and enzyme and hormone action. Calcium is an important intracellular messenger, which has an essential role in the maintenance of cell membrane potential of nerve and cardiac cells and contractile muscle cells. It is absorbed by active transport in the duodenum. Total body calcium is about 1–2 kg with 99% held in the skeleton, 1% intracellular and 0.1% extracellular.

The average level of calcium in plasma is 2.5 mmol/L, but levels range from 2.2–2.6 mmol/L. A level of > 2.6 mmol/L, taking into account corrected levels, would indicate a state of hypercalcaemia. In hypoalbuminaemia, there is less calcium in the bound state and therefore a higher level of total calcium.

72. A　Bone metastases

Bone is the third most common site of metastases. Five cancers most frequently metastasising to bone are breast, lung, prostate, thyroid and kidney. Consequences include pain, pathological fractures and hypercalcaemia. Pain results from stretching of the periosteum and stimulation of nerves in the endosteum. Lytic lesions of bones lead to pathological fractures. Multiple myeloma is a cancer of plasma cells. Proliferation of plasma cells interferes with normal production of blood cells within the bone marrow, resulting in anaemia, leucopenia and thrombocytopaenia. Patients develop hypercalcaemia in this condition due to excessive tumour-induced osteoclast-mediated bone destruction, caused by cytokines expressed or secreted locally at myeloma cells. This leads to an efflux of calcium into the extracellular fluid.

73. E　PTH acts via a G-protein coupled receptor

Parathyroid hormone (PTH) acts to increase circulating levels of calcium and phosphate. It acts via a G-protein coupled receptor. In the kidney, PTH acts proximally at the renal tubules to increase bicarbonate and phosphate excretion. At the distal renal tubule, calcium and hydrogen are reabsorbed in response to PTH action. Alpha1-hydroxylation of vitamin D takes place in the kidney and this is enhanced by PTH action. PTH enhances the osteoclastic activity in bone, enhancing bone resorption.

PTH acts on many organ systems:

- Bone: PTH increases release of calcium, indirectly stimulates osteoclasts, and increases bone resorption
- Kidney: PTH enhances active reabsorption of calcium and magnesium from distal tubules, increases excretion of phosphate
- Intestine: PTH increases absorption of calcium by increasing production of vitamin D

74. A　Active transport

Calcium and phosphate are transferred to the fetal circulation against a concentration by active transport. The fetus is relatively hypercalcaemic compared to the mother at a ratio of 1:1.4 and contains approximately 21–33 g of calcium. Ossification occurs mainly in the third trimester, when the majority of the calcium accumulates. Active transport also facilitates the transfer of substances such as amino acids across the placenta. Substances such as oxygen and carbon dioxide travel via passive diffusion across a concentration gradient, whereas transport molecules aid the transfer of substances such as glucose in the form of facilitated diffusion.

75. A　Increased calcitonin

During pregnancy and breastfeeding the female body has an increased requirement for calcium. The fetus is hypercalcaemic compared to the mother and most of the calcium reserve in the fetus is attained during the third trimester. The fetus is able to produce parathyroid hormone at around 12 weeks' gestation. During pregnancy, the mother has a reduced level of parathyroid hormone and an increased level of calcitonin in order to maintain an increased transfer of calcium to the fetus. There is an overall increase in bone turnover during the third trimester.

76. A The number of deaths during the first 28 completed days of life per 1000 live births

The World Health Organization defines the neonatal mortality rate as the number of deaths during the first 28 completed days of life per 1000 live births in a given year or period. It considers the neonatal period to begin at birth and to carry on until 28 completed days of life. The definition includes babies who have shown any sign of life following delivery, even if this is only for a short period of time.

77. A The proportion of women with a normal pregnancy who had a low-risk result

The specificity of a test is its ability to correctly identify those individuals without any pathology, so in this case, it refers to the proportion of women who had a normal pregnancy and were given a correct low-risk result at screening. The specificity of a test should aim to be as high as possible, i.e. as close to 1 or 100% as possible.

The sensitivity of a test is its ability to correctly identify affected/high risk individuals. For this test it is the proportion of women with an affected fetus who were given a high-risk result at screening. The sensitivity of a test should also aim to be as close to 1 or 100% as possible.

78. B 0.2

The standard error of the mean (SEM) is a measure of how close the sample mean lies from the mean of the true population. The larger the sample size (n), the smaller the SEM, and the smaller the SEM, the more accurate an estimate the sample mean is of the true population mean. The SEM can be calculated using only the sample size and the standard deviation.

SEM = Standard deviation $\div \sqrt{n}$

Standard deviation = 2, n = 100
SEM = $2 \div \sqrt{n}$
    = $2 \div 10$
    = 0.2

79. B Cohort study

The research study described has used a cohort study design. Within this design subjects from the exposure group (in this case maternal smoking) and the non-exposure group can be followed over a long period of time. This type of study is time-consuming as any differences between the two groups may take a long time to surface. Cohort studies may be subject to bias and confounding variables, but they have the potential to provide an immense amount of detail about the study groups over a long period and therefore give the opportunity to realise unexpected outcomes. They may have either a retrospective or prospective design, and in this case, there is the potential to employ a retrospective design based on hospital notes.

80. B The erroneous rejection of the null hypothesis

In order to understand type 1 and type 2 errors it is essential to understand what is meant by the null hypothesis. The null hypothesis must be defined before any statistical analysis takes place. The standard null hypothesis states that there is no difference between the sample groups being looked at. A type 1 error (also known as an α error) is said to have occurred in a study when the null hypothesis has been wrongly rejected. In simpler terms the study has reported a difference that does not exist.

A type 2 error (also known as a β error) is actually more common than a type 1 error and is said to have occurred when the null hypothesis has been accepted when there is, in fact, a difference between the sample groups being looked at.

81. D Community-acquired Group A streptococcal disease

The 'Mothers and Babies: Reducing Risk through Audits and Confidential Enquiries across the UK' (MBRRACE-UK) programme classifies causes of maternal mortality as directly related, indirectly related or coincidental to pregnancy. Directly related causes of maternal mortality are those that result from obstetric complications. In the options A to E, the only cause directly related to pregnancy is community-acquired group A streptococcal disease. Genital tract sepsis, predominantly due to group A streptococcal disease, was given as the leading direct cause of maternal death in the report, and its incidence had increased since the previous triennial report. Causes of death that are indirectly related to pregnancy are those that are not caused by obstetric complications but were made worse by the physiological changes associated with pregnancy. These indirectly related causes include conditions that were pre-existing or were diagnosed during pregnancy.

Within the UK, suicide is included as one of the indirectly related causes of maternal death because it is usually the result of puerperal psychosis. Other indirect causes include cardiac disease, diabetes and hormone-dependent cancers.

Knight M, Kenyon S, Brocklehurst P, Neilson J, Shakespeare J, Kurinczuk JJ (Eds.) on behalf of MBRRACEUK. Saving Lives, Improving Mothers' Care - Lessons learned to inform future maternity care from the UK and Ireland Confidential Enquiries into Maternal Deaths and Morbidity 2009–12. Oxford: National Perinatal Epidemiology Unit, University of Oxford 2014.

82. B The middle value in a ranked set of data

The median is one of the terms used to describe an 'average' of a set of data. The median is the middle value in a ranked data set. It should not be confused with the mode, which refers to the most frequently occurring value in a data set. It also differs from the mean, which is calculated by dividing the sum of a data set by the number of values in the data set. An advantage of using the median is that it is uninfluenced by outliers or skewed data, which can affect the mean of a data set. The median figure in a data set may be higher or lower than the mean.

83. D Patau's syndrome

Patau's syndrome is also known as trisomy 13. This condition is less common than trisomy 18 or trisomy 21. Patau's syndrome occurs when there is an extra copy of chromosome 13. This extra chromosome usually arises after a non-disjunction event during meiosis, however it can also occur as a result of a Robertsonian translocation. More rarely an individual may be mosaic for trisomy 13, i.e. only some of their cells will be trisomy 13, whereas other cells have a normal complement of chromosomes.

High-risk antenatal screening results may be suggestive of a trisomy, and can be confirmed by subsequent invasive testing, such as amniocentesis. An affected fetus generally has multiple organ system defects. Common abnormalities include microcephaly, polydactyly, bilateral cleft palate and cardiac defects. The majority of babies born with Patau's syndrome die within the first month of life, and few survive infancy.

84. E 47 XXY

This boy has Klinefelter's syndrome, which is a relatively common disorder of the sex chromosomes. Around 1 in every 1000 male babies born have Klinefelter's syndrome. Affected individuals typically have the genotype 47 XXY, indicating that they have an extra X chromosome. This extra chromosome is present due a non-disjunction event in either spermatogenesis or oogenesis. Physical features associated with Klinefelter's syndrome include above average height, long arms and legs, gynaecomastia, a female body fat distribution and varying development of secondary sexual characteristics. Undiagnosed individuals typically present due to concern regarding gynaecomastia or unexplained infertility. Historically, individuals with Klinefelter's syndrome have been described as experiencing higher levels of behavioural difficulties and having lower IQs than average, although these stereotypes are probably unjustified.

85. D Mosaic for Down's syndrome

The karyotype given informs us that some of the fetus' cells are of the karyotype 46 XX, whereas other cells detected have an extra chromosome 21 and therefore contain 47 chromosomes (hence described as 47 XX + 21). This unusual finding is called mosaicism and refers to the existence of two different cell lines within an individual, each with a different number of chromosomes.

Mosaicism is most commonly caused by a non-disjunction event occurring during an early embryonic mitotic division, which leaves some cells with an uneven number of chromosomes; i.e. some cells have a trisomy, whereas others have a normal number of chromosomes. The presence of mosaicism in fetuses is diagnosed by amniocentesis or chorionic villi sampling with analysis typically describing the percentage of cells with a normal karyotype versus those of a different cell line. Mosaicism is only found in 1% of cases of Down's syndrome. As the proportion of cells with trisomy 21 varies it is difficult to predict to what extent the individual will be affected.

86. D Marfan's syndrome

Marfan's syndrome is a connective tissue disorder is caused by a mutation in the FBN1 gene found on chromosome 15 that codes for the protein fibrillin-1. It is an autosomal dominant condition, however in some affected individuals the gene mutation has occurred de novo. The individual described has the characteristic appearance of Marfan's syndrome. In addition to tall stature, long arms and digits, people with Marfan's syndrome may also have scoliosis and deformities of the chest wall. This individual has known aortic root dilation, a common finding in many affected individuals. Other cardiac sequelae include aortic dissection and mitral valve prolapse.

Congenital contractual arachnodactyly is an autosomal dominant condition causing skeletal abnormalities as a consequence of a mutation of the protein fibrillin-2. Ehlers–Danlos syndrome refers to heterogenous group of disorders associated with defects in collagen synthesis, the classical form of which is an autosomal dominant inherited condition.

87. E Leber's optic neuropathy

The mitochondria contain their own DNA (mtDNA), which is transmitted from a mother to her children. In humans there are 37 genes contained within mitochondrial DNA. Although both male and female offspring may be affected by any inherited mutations in mtDNA, only females can pass these defects onto the next generation. Leber's optic neuropathy is transmitted by mitochondrial inheritance. As mitochondria are key to cellular oxidative phosphorylation, mutations in mitochondrial DNA tend to manifest in systems heavily reliant on this process. Hence mitochondrial disease tends to manifest as a myopathy. Leber's optic neuropathy is one such condition and is caused by three known mutations of mitochondrial DNA. Colour blindness and Duchenne muscular dystrophy are both X-linked recessive conditions. Dermatomyositis is an autoimmune connective tissue disease. Alpha-thalassaemia is an autosomal recessive condition.

88. A Angelman's syndrome

Genomic imprinting refers to the loss of either a maternal or paternal allele. It is known that maternally and paternally derived alleles are not the same, and there can be devastating results if an allele is inactivated. Both Angelman's syndrome and Prader–Willi syndrome are examples of genomic imprinting with deleterious effects. In Angelman's syndrome there is loss of area of the long arm of the maternally derived chromosome 15, whereas Prader–Willi syndrome is caused by loss of the same area of the paternally derived chromosome. The syndromes are distinct but both are associated with mental retardation. It is of note that genomic imprinting (i.e. the inactivation of one parent's copy of a gene) does occur naturally without harmful effect. Both Fragile-X syndrome and Friedreich ataxia are examples of trinucleotide repeat disorders. Patau's syndrome is caused by trisomy of chromosome 13.

89. C Oxytocin

As well as transporting molecules between the mother and the fetus, the placenta functions as an important endocrine organ during pregnancy. It synthesises and secretes many hormones, which function to maintain and support the pregnancy.

It synthesises and secretes two major types of hormones: steroid hormones (progesterone and oestrogen) and protein hormones [human chorionic gonadotropin (hCG), relaxin and human placental lactogen].

The syncytiotrophoblast cells of the placenta secrete hCG, progesterone and oestrogen. The placental lactogens are thought to be involved in mobilising energy stores for the fetus. Relaxin works synergistically with progesterone in maintaining the pregnancy. Oxytocin is secreted by the posterior pituitary gland and is not produced by the placenta.

90. D Umbilical arteries arise from the internal iliac artery

The umbilical cord contains three vessels: two arteries and one vein. These vessels are contained in Wharton's jelly. The cord is formed at 5 weeks' gestation and at term has a mean length of 50 cm and width of 2 cm. The umbilical arteries arise from the internal iliac artery and the veins drain mainly into the inferior vena cava (80%) via the ductus venosus and 20% into the hepatic vein. 1% of umbilical cords have a single artery and of this 1%, 20% will have a cardiovascular abnormality. Other abnormalities of the cord include knots, which may be false or true. False knots are unusual vascular structures and true knots are more common in longer cords. Velamentous cord insertion describes the situation, where the umbilical cord inserts into the chorioamniotic membranes rather than the mass of the placenta. These vessels are therefore not protected in part by Wharton's jelly. This is associated with vasa praevia.

91. A Active transport: amino acids

The placenta supplies the growing fetus with oxygen and nutrients, as well as providing a means for the removal of carbon dioxide and other waste products and metabolites. The movement of these substances is largely dictated by their size and occurs through passive diffusion, active transport and facilitated diffusion, in addition to exocytosis and endocytosis.

Transport across the placenta:

- Passive diffusion: oxygen, carbon dioxide, free fatty acids, urea
- Active transport: amino acids

- Facilitated diffusion: glucose
- Receptor mediated endocytosis: IgG

92. E Vasodilation

Oestrogen exerts a series of effects, both at local and systemic levels. Oestrogen promotes vascular tone, leading to vasodilation, with both rapid and chronic effect. There are two oestrogen receptors: α and β. The α-receptor is found on the endothelial cell membrane and directly activates nitric oxide. Oestrogen is involved in other systemic changes, e.g. it helps maintain bone density levels, increases clotting and decreases cholesterol and low-density lipoprotein levels. Other properties include protection against atherosclerosis.

93. B It contains 154 mmol/L sodium chloride

0.9% normal saline is a crystalloid solution and contains 154 mmol/L sodium chloride. It has an osmolarity of 308 mOsmol/L and does not contain any potassium chloride. There is, however, the capacity to add potassium chloride to the fluid if there is an indication to replace these electrolytes, e.g. gastric loss. It mainly replaces the extracellular fluid component of body water and only a quarter of the volume replaced will make it into the plasma.

Colloids are better volume expanders than crystalloid fluids as they remain in the intravascular compartment for a longer period.

Postoperatively, there is a sympathoadrenal stress response. This may lead to an increase in the retention of sodium and water as a result of increased antidiuretic hormone secretion and therefore the use of saline may not be the most appropriate fluid to use.

94. B The fetus loses metabolites to the mother

The Bohr effect describes a situation where an increase in carbon dioxide in the blood and a decrease in pH leads to a reduction in the affinity for oxygen.

The double Bohr effect refers to the situation in the maternal–fetal circulation where the Bohr effect is operative on both sides. This improves the oxygen transfer between mother and fetus.

Maternal:

- Reduced pH
- Oxygen curve shift to right
- Reduced affinity to oxygen
- Uptake of fetal metabolites

Fetal:

- Increased pH
- Oxygen curve shift to left
- Increased affinity to oxygen
- Loss of metabolites to maternal circulation

95. C Two alpha chains and two gamma chains (α2γ2)

Fetal haemoglobin (HbF) is the predominant form of haemoglobin present in fetal life and consists of four chains, α2 and γ2. HbF replaces embryonic haemoglobin after around 10 weeks' gestation and is present in high levels throughout gestation. Adult haemoglobin (HbA) has α2 chains and two β2 chains. HbA is also present in small amounts from the first trimester, but production starts to increase in the third trimester in preparation of ex-utero life. At birth HbF represents at least 50% of the haemoglobin present, but by 6 months of age this has been replaced by adult haemoglobin. Unlike adult haemoglobin, HbF does not bind with 2,3-diphosphoglycerate (2,3-DPG). As a consequence HbF has a higher affinity for oxygen than adult haemoglobin, allowing oxygen to dissociate from maternal haemoglobin and be transferred to the fetal circulation across the placenta. With a higher affinity for oxygen than adult haemoglobin, the dissociation curve for HbF sits to the left of that of adult haemoglobin. The dissociation curve illustrates that with its higher affinity for oxygen HbF becomes saturated with oxygen at lower partial pressures than HbA.

96. B Luteinising hormone

The luteinising hormone surge (LH) instigates a series of steps that lead to ovulation. During the follicular phase of the menstrual cycle the level of LH slowly increases. The dominant follicle expresses LH receptors leading to increasing amounts of oestradiol production by the theca cells (due to the conversion of cholesterol). This elevated level of oestrogen instigates a positive feedback response by LH with a subsequent surge at around day 14. This surge leads to the extrusion of the oocyte from the follicle. After release of the oocyte, LH supports the corpus luteum, formed from the disrupted granulosa and thecal cells, to produce progesterone and oestradiol.

97. D At fertilisation

Oogenesis is the process where an ovum is formed in females from primordial germ cells. The primordial germ cells develop in the fetal gonadal tissue, which eventually becomes the fetal ovary, and the primordial germ cells become oogonia. The oogonia undergo division by mitosis, rapidly increasing in number to form several million oogonia by the second trimester of fetal life. Oogonia then become primary oocytes through mitosis. Surrounded by primordial follicles, the primary oocytes are diploid; they begin meiosis 1 during the third trimester of pregnancy, and this is arrested at prophase. They remain in this state until ovulation many years later. At ovulation, meiosis 1 recommences leading to the production of the secondary oocyte and the first polar body. The secondary oocyte is haploid and immediately after meiosis 1 is completed enters meiosis 2. This second meiotic division becomes halted at metaphase II. The second meiotic division, leading to the production of a mature ovum and the second polar body, is only completed should fertilisation occur.

98. B Inferior vena cava

The ductus venosus acts as one of the three fetal circulatory shunts, in addition to the ductus arteriosus and the foramen ovale. The ductus venosus is the blood vessel that runs from the umbilical vein and communicates with the inferior vena cava (IVC). This shunt allows much of the fetal oxygenated blood supply to bypass the liver, with preferential distribution to the brain. The ductus venosus starts to close soon after birth. In adults the remnant of the ductus venosus is known as the ligamentum venosum. The fetal umbilical vein eventually becomes the ligamentum teres. The passage between the fetal left and right atria is known as the foramen ovale. Blood passes through the foramen ovale from the right atria to the left atria. The foramen ovale closes soon after birth and eventually becomes the fossa ovalis. Failure of the foramen ovale to close is not uncommon and in the majority of individuals the persistence of this shunt remains undiagnosed. It has been suggested that a patent foramen ovale may be associated with unexplained transient ischaemic events and migraines.

99. D Superior gluteal artery

The internal iliac artery is the main artery of the pelvic organs and also the perineum. The internal iliac artery begins at the bifurcation of the common iliac artery. It then divides into anterior and posterior branches. The branches of the anterior division of the internal iliac artery predominantly supply the pelvic organs, i.e. the uterus, vagina, bladder, lower part of the rectum as well as several muscles of the buttocks. The superior gluteal artery is a branch of the posterior division of the internal iliac artery (**Tables 15.6** and **15.7**). Note the ovarian artery supplies the ovaries, which is a branch of the abdominal aorta.

Table 15.6 Major branches of the internal iliac artery

Artery	Female organs and muscles supplied
Umbilical	Superior part of urinary bladder
Obturator	Femoral head, ilium, muscles of medial thigh, pelvic muscles
Uterine	Uterus, fallopian tubes, vagina, uterine ligaments
Internal pudendal	Perineum, anal canal, external genitalia
Middle rectal	Lower part of rectum
Inferior gluteal	Pelvic diaphragm

Table 15.7 Major branches of the posterior iliac artery

Artery	Organ
Iliolumbar	Muscles of posterior abdominal walls, i.e. quadrates lumborum, iliacus and psoas major
	Cauda equina
Lateral sacral arteries (superior and inferior)	Piriformis, erector spinae, sacral canal
Superior gluteal	Gluteus minimus
	Gluteus maximus
	Gluteus medius
	Tensor fascia lata
	Piriformis

100. B Iliacus

The iliacus muscle does not form part of the anterior abdominal wall and is innervated by the femoral nerve. The anterior abdominal wall provides support for the internal structures. The muscles of the anterior abdominal wall are:

- Rectus abdominis – from costal cartilages to the pubic crest
- Pyramidalis – may be absent (1 in 5 individuals), lies anterior to lower fibres of rectus abdominis
- External oblique – runs downwards and forwards from large insertion from lower 8th ribs
- Internal oblique – runs opposite to the external oblique, upwards and forwards from anterior iliac crest and inguinal ligament

Chapter 16

Mock Paper 2

The 100 single best answers presented in this chapter should be worked through under exam conditions and completed in two and a half hours.

Questions

For each question, select the single best answer from the five options listed.

1. What range of wave frequencies is used in ultrasonography?

   A 0.5–1 MHz
   B 1–20 MHz
   C 30–50 MHz
   D 50–100 MHz
   E 100 MHz

2. A 32-year-old woman is para 1 and is seen in the antenatal clinic at 36 weeks' gestation to discuss the mode of delivery. Her last labour resulted in an emergency caesarean section at 8 cm dilatation for fetal distress. You are counselling her about the risks of vaginal birth after caesarean section (VBAC).

   What risk of uterine rupture should be quoted to patients when counselling about VBAC?

   A 1 in 100
   B 1 in 200
   C 1 in 500
   D 1 in 1000
   E 1 in 2000

3. A 28-year-old multiparous woman attends for a dating scan in early pregnancy. She is unsure of the first day of her last menstrual period and reports that her periods are irregular. Fetal heart activity is detected on the transvaginal scan.

   What is the earliest gestation that fetal heart action can be detected on a transvaginal ultrasound scan?

   A 3–4 weeks
   B 4–5 weeks
   C 5–6 weeks
   D 6–7 weeks
   E 7–8 weeks

4. A 40-year-old multiparous woman is 32 weeks pregnant. She reports recurrent palpitations. Her general practitioner arranges for her to have an electrocardiogram (ECG).

   Which of the following features of a standard ECG represents ventricular depolarisation?

   A P-wave
   B PR interval
   C QRS complex
   D QT interval
   E T wave

5. A 33-year-old woman with HIV is seen in a genitourinary clinic. She has not commenced antiretroviral therapy. She describes deep dyspareunia, bilateral pelvic pain and increased vaginal discharge. She is otherwise well and is apyrexial. Serum inflammatory markers are normal. She is treated for suspected pelvic inflammatory disease.

   What is the most appropriate treatment?

   A An extended course of oral antibiotics for 1 month
   B Initiation of antiretrovirals
   C Inpatient treatment for intravenous antibiotics
   D Standard 2 weeks of antibiotic treatment
   E None of the above

6. A 27-year-old woman presents at 26 weeks' gestation with a 2-day history of painful genital lesions. She does not recall having had any previous episodes. On examination, she has labial vesicles, which are tender to touch. She is diagnosed with genital herpes.

   What is the most appropriate management?

   A Arrange for an elective caesarean section at 37 weeks' gestation
   B Counsel the woman regarding termination of pregnancy
   C Organise ultrasound scans every 4 weeks for the remainder of the pregnancy
   D Referral to a genitourinary physician for treatment in line with her condition
   E None of the above

7. A 32-year-old woman presents with a 7-year history of painful periods, and a 3-year history of primary subfertility. Her serum follicular-stimulating hormone level is 6.8 IU/mL and luteinising hormone is 6.7 IU/mL. Pelvic ultrasound was unremarkable and her partner's semen analysis was normal.

   What is the most appropriate investigation in this woman?

   A Laparoscopy and dye test
   B Brain MRI to exclude a prolactinoma
   C Postcoital test
   D Serum anti-Müllerian hormone levels
   E Serum testosterone level

8. A 40-year-old woman at 28-weeks' gestation presents to the delivery suit with a 4-hour history of absent fetal movements and abdominal pain. On examination, she is pale and has a hard tender abdomen. There is no fetal heart audible.

What is the most appropriate immediate plan of management?

   A Administer corticosteroids
   B Category one caesarean section
   C Induction of labour with prostaglandins
   D Intravenous access and resuscitation
   E Magnesium sulphate infusion

9. A 41-year-old grand multiparous woman has a vaginal delivery. The midwife reports that she felt dizzy and has now collapsed in a pool of blood while walking to the toilet.

What is the most appropriate initial management?

   A Call for immediate help
   B Cannulate the patient and send blood for a cross match
   C Ensure her placenta is complete
   D Prescribe 40 IU oxytocin over 4 hours
   E Catheterise the patient as her bladder is palpable

10. A 25-year-old primiparous woman who is currently at 35 weeks' gestation is seen at a routine antenatal clinic. Her body mass index at booking was 23 kg/m². Her blood pressure is 110/62 mmHg. She has moderate ankle oedema and is worried she has pre-eclampsia.

Which action is the most appropriate?

   A Admit to hospital
   B Assess serum transaminase levels
   C Re-check her blood pressure in 30 minutes
   D Perform a urine dipstick to assess for proteinuria
   E Start antihypertensives immediately

11. A 32-year-old woman is admitted to hospital 10 days after a first trimester miscarriage. She complains of abdominal pain, increased vaginal bleeding and offensive smelling discharge. An ultrasound scan reveals evidence of retained products of conception of 45 × 50 × 37 mm.

What is the most appropriate management?

   A Evacuation of retained products of conception (ERPC)
   B Intravenous antibiotics
   C Intravenous antibiotics followed by an ERPC
   D Oral antibiotics and repeat ultrasound scan in 2 days
   E Repeat ultrasound scan in 2 weeks

12. A 39-year-old woman attends the gynaecology clinic complaining of increasingly irregular menstrual cycles, mood swings and weight gain. Hormone profile shows the following:

Follicle-stimulating hormone	32 IU/L
Luteinising hormone	4 IU/L
Oestradiol	52 IU/L
Prolactin	215 mIU/L
Thyroid function tests	Normal

What is the most likely diagnosis?

A   Asherman's syndrome
B   Addison's disease
C   Polycystic ovarian syndrome
D   Pregnancy
E   Premature ovarian failure

13. A 33-year-old woman attends the gynaecology clinic for investigation of her recurrent first trimester miscarriages. A thrombophilia screen has been performed as part of routine investigation.

Which of the following positive results would most likely suggest an acquired thrombophilia, rather than an inherited one?

A   Activated protein C resistance
B   Anticardiolipin antibodies
C   Antithrombin III deficiency
D   Protein C deficiency
E   Protein S deficiency

14. A 32-year-old woman attends for a review at 28 weeks' gestation. She complains of a circular rash on her legs and mild shortness of breath. Chest X-ray reveals bilateral hilar lymphadenopathy. Her blood tests show a mildly elevated serum angiotensin-converting enzyme level.

What is the most likely diagnosis?

A   Crohn's disease
B   Polyarteritis nodosa
C   Sarcoidosis
D   Tuberculosis
E   Wegener's granulomatosis

15. A multiparous woman is in spontaneous labour at 40 weeks' gestation. She has had one previous caesarean section. She is being continuously monitored in labour using cardiotocography (CTG). Her midwife is concerned that the CTG shows reduced beat-to-beat variability.

Regarding CTG analysis, what is considered the normal range for beat-to-beat variability?

A   5–25 beats per minute
B   2–8 beats per minute
C   5–10 beats per minute

D   5–15 beats per minute
E   10–25 beats per minute

16. A 23-year-old woman attends her 16-week antenatal appointment. Her booking blood tests for hepatitis serology are as follows:

HBsAg	Positive
Anti-HBc	Positive
Anti-HBs	Negative
Anti-HBc IgM	Negative

What is the patient's most likely hepatitis B status?

A   Acute infection
B   Chronic infection
C   Previous immunisation
D   Resolving acute infection
E   Susceptible to hepatitis B infection

17. A 29-year-old hirsute woman attends the gynaecology outpatient clinic. She has oligomenorrhea and secondary subfertility. Her ultrasound scan shows ovaries with multiple peripheral cysts.

What is her anti-Müllerian hormone profile most likely to be?

A   Undetectable
B   3.7 pmol/L
C   10 pmol/L
D   17.3 pmol/L
E   65 pmol/L

18. A nulliparous woman has an early pregnancy ultrasound scan. Her serum human chorionic gonadotropin (hCG) level is taken as part of a study looking at the correlation between gestational age and serum hCG levels. The scan shows a single ongoing intrauterine pregnancy at 7 weeks' gestation.

Which is the most likely serum hCG level to correspond with this pregnancy?

A   50 IU/L
B   120 IU/L
C   300 IU/L
D   5000 IU/L
E   300,000 IU/L

19. Type III hypersensitivity reactions occur in which of the following conditions?

A   Goodpasture syndrome
B   Multiple sclerosis
C   Rheumatoid arthritis
D   Streptococcal nephritis
E   Tuberculosis

20. Which of the following immunoglobulin isotopes crosses the placenta to give the fetus passive immunity?

    A IgA
    B IgD
    C IgE
    D IgG
    E IgM

21. Which of the following is a major function of the complement system?

    A Acquisition of fetal immunity
    B Hypersensitivity
    C Opsonisation
    D Pyknosis
    E Sensitisation

22. A 37-year-old woman is seen in the gynaecology outpatient clinic complaining of a profuse, fishy-smelling, thin grey vaginal discharge; microscopy shows the presence of clue cells; the whiff test is positive.

    Which is the most likely causative agent?

    A *Candida albicans*
    B *Chlamydia trachomatis*
    C *Gardnerella vaginalis*
    D *Escherichia coli*
    E *Trichomonas vaginalis*

23. A 35-year-old nulliparous woman is 14 weeks pregnant. She has recently arrived in the United Kingdom from a South American country. She is under the care of the infectious diseases team who are concerned she has yaws.

    Which of the following is the cause of yaws?

    A *Treponema pallidum carateum*
    B *Treponema pallidum endemicum*
    C *Treponema pallidum pallidum*
    D *Treponema pallidum pertenue*
    E *Treponema paraluis cuniculi*

24. A 25-year-old nulliparous woman is being seen in a fetal medicine clinic following the detection of hydrops fetalis at a routine anomaly scan. Following investigation primary maternal cytomegalovirus infection is suspected.

    Which of the options below gives the genome structure for cytomegalovirus (CMV)?

    A dsDNA
    B ssDNA
    C dsRNA
    D dsDNA-RT
    E ssRNA-RT

25. A 53-year-old woman undergoes a total abdominal hysterectomy and bilateral salpingo-oophorectomy after an ovarian mass was discovered on MRI. Her body mass index is 38 kg/m² and postoperative recovery is delayed by a suspected wound infection. Three days postoperatively, she has a temperature of 38.1°C, heart rate of 110 beats per minute and blood pressure of 94/56 mmHg. On examination, her wound is erythematous with serosanguineous exudate.

What is the most likely cause?

A   *Escherichia coli*
B   *Proteus*
C   *Pseudomonas aeruginosa*
D   *Staphylococcus aureus*
E   *Streptococcus pyogenes*

26. A 26-year-old woman undergoes a grade one emergency caesarean section for fetal bradycardia. She has diabetes and is obese. Ten days after the operation, she is readmitted with a wound infection. The wound is erythematous and discharging pus. There were no intraoperative complications.

What is the most likely operative factor contributing to the infection?

A   Length of operation
B   Presence of foreign material at operative site
C   Sterility of instruments
D   Surgical technique
E   Underlying medical disorder

27. A 19-year-old woman has attended her local genitourinary medicine clinic for a sexual health screening. Routine vaginal and endocervical swabs are taken and show the presence of a Gram-negative bacterium. A diagnosis of *Neisseria gonorrhoeae* is made. The presence of which bacterial cell component is detected by the Gram stain?

A   Glycocalyx
B   Mycolic acid
C   N-acetyl glucosamine
D   N-acetyl muramic acid
E   Peptidoglycan

28. A woman attends the emergency department with severe left iliac fossa pain and a small amount of vaginal bleeding. On examination, her abdomen is distended with guarding and rebound tenderness. A urine pregnancy test is positive. An urgent transvaginal scan shows a left tubal ectopic pregnancy.

Which of the following is a recognised risk factor for ectopic pregnancy?

A   Combined oral contraceptive pill usage
B   Multiparity
C   Obesity
D   Smoking
E   Young maternal age

29. Which of the following is typical of acute inflammation?

   A   Angiogenesis
   B   Centralisation of leucocytes
   C   Decreased capillary hydrostatic pressure
   D   Increased efficiency of axial blood flow
   E   Increased endothelial permeability

30. Which of the following is a site of primary choriocarcinoma occurrence?

   A   Liver
   B   Lungs
   C   Testicles
   D   Thyroid
   E   Urinary bladder

31. A 40-year-old woman primiparous woman has an emergency caesarean section at 36 weeks' gestation following the onset of severe pre-eclampsia. After delivery the placenta is sent for histological analysis.

Which of the following is a histological change seen in the placenta in pre-eclampsia?

   A   Decreased syncytial knots
   B   Fibrosed villi
   C   Mass of small capillaries
   D   Non-specific trophoblast hyperplasia
   E   Villous hypovascularity with evidence of infarction

32. A 26-year-old nulliparous woman attends a colposcopy clinic following an abnormal smear test. A biopsy taken at colposcopy shows dysplasic changes typical of cervical intraepithelial neoplasia.

Which of the following is a histological change seen in dysplasia?

   A   Increased nuclear size
   B   Increased number of cells
   C   Hyperchromatism
   D   Presence of meiotic figures
   E   Reduction in cell size

33. Which of the following is a cause of pregnancy-related microangiopathic haemolytic anaemia?

   A   Disseminated intravascular coagulopathy
   B   Gestational diabetes
   C   Polymorphic eruption of pregnancy
   D   Pregnancy-induced hypertension
   E   Pregnancy-induced idiopathic thrombocytopaenic purpura

34. A 53-year-old woman is brought to the emergency department by ambulance. She had a total abdominal hysterectomy and bilateral salpingo-oophorectomy 7 days ago and is in extremis. She is clearly unwell and the doctors treating her suspect she has systemic inflammatory response syndrome.

Which of the following is one of the diagnostic criteria of SIRS?

A   Heart rate > 75 beats per minute
B $Paco_2$ > 6.3 kPa
C   Respiratory rate > 15 breaths per minute
D   Temperature > 37.5°C
E   White cell count < 4 × 10^9 cells/L

35. Which of the following hormones is secreted by the acidophils of the anterior pituitary gland?

A   Adrenocorticotrophic hormone
B   Follicle-stimulating hormone
C   Growth hormone
D   Oxytocin
E   Thyroid-stimulating hormone

36. What is the most common type of pituitary adenoma?

A   Adrenocorticotrophic hormone-secreting adenoma
B   Growth hormone-secreting adenoma
C   Prolactin-secreting adenoma
D   Mammosomatotroph adenoma
E   Mixed growth hormone/prolactin-secreting adenoma

37. Which of the following is a premalignant condition?

A   Erythroplakia
B   Herpes simplex infection
C   Lichen sclerosus
D   Lichen planus
E   Pemphigus vulgaris

38. Which of the following is a recognised risk factor for the development of cervical cancer?

A   Early menarche
B   Higher socioeconomic status
C   Early age of first sexual intercourse
D   Having a male partner who has been circumcised
E   Use of the oral contraceptive pill

39. A 56-year-old woman attends the gynaecology outpatient clinic with a history of postmenopausal bleeding. A pelvic ultrasound shows an endometrial thickness of 8 mm. Following an endometrial Pipelle biopsy and an MRI, a diagnosis of stage 1a endometrial cancer is made.

Which of the following is a risk factor for the development of endometrial cancer?

A   History of endometriosis
B   Multiparity
C   Non-hormonal intrauterine device (IUD) usage
D   Obesity
E   Premature menopause

40. A 27-year-old woman has a smear test as part of the UK screening programme. Following an abnormal result she attends a colposcopy clinic. A sample is taken during the colposcopy and sent for human papilloma virus (HPV) typing.

Which of the following HPV subtypes is high-risk for the development of cervical intraepithelial neoplasia?

A   HPV 2
B   HPV 6
C   HPV 11
D   HPV 16
E   HPV 63

41. Which receptor is responsible for the analgesic effect of morphine?

A   Acetylcholine
B δ
C   k
D μ
E   N-methyl-d-aspartate (NMDA) receptor

42. A 42-year-old woman delivers a baby at term weighing 2.5 kg. The baby is found to have abnormalities including chondrodysplasia and hypoplasia of the nasal bridge.

Which medication is most likely to have caused these abnormalities?

A   Azathioprine
B   Chloramphenicol
C   Gentamicin
D   Sodium valproate
E   Warfarin

43. What is the mechanism of action of warfarin?

A   Activation of antithrombin III
B   Increases action of factor Xa
C   Increases production of factors II, VII, IX and X
D   Increases production of vitamin K
E   Inhibits enzymic reduction of vitamin K

44. A 24-year-old woman undergoes a grade 1 caesarean section under general anaesthetic.

What is the most appropriate induction agent that should be used?

A   Etomidate
B   Ketamine
C   Midazolam
D   Propofol
E   Thiopental

45. A 16-year-old primiparous is seen on the postnatal ward round 3 days after delivery. She wishes to discuss contraception, as this pregnancy was unplanned and she leads a hectic lifestyle. She is breastfeeding.

What is the most appropriate contraception?

A   Condoms
B   Progesterone-only subdermal implant
C   Combined oral contraceptive pill
D   Diaphragm
E   Progesterone-only contraceptive pill

46. A 19-year-old woman who is 28 weeks pregnant requests treatment for acne and is prescribed an antibiotic by her general practitioner (GP). She goes on to deliver a healthy baby girl at term. Two years later her daughter is noted to have unusually grey teeth.

Which treatment for acne did her GP prescribed for acne?

A   Chloramphenicol
B   Cefalexin
C   Co-trimoxazole
D   Erythromycin
E   Oxytetracycline

47. A 36-year-old woman with essential hypertension is 5 weeks pregnant. Prior to pregnancy she was taking an antihypertensive that has been associated with the development of fetal renal defects and oligohydramnios.

Which antihypertensive was she taking?

A   Atenolol
B   Labetalol
C   Methyldopa
D   Nifedipine
E   Ramipril

48. A 25-year-old nulliparous woman with a lifelong history of tonic-clonic seizures sees her neurologist for advice as she wishes to start a family.

Which anticonvulsant drug is the most potentially teratogenic?

A   Carbamazepine
B   Lamotrigine

    C   Levetiracetam

    D   Phenytoin

    E   Sodium valproate

49. A 21-year-old woman presents to the emergency department with vaginal spotting and mild lower abdominal pain. She has a positive pregnancy test and serum human chorionic gonadotrophin is 2562 IU/L. She is found to have evidence of a left tubal ectopic pregnancy on pelvic ultrasound scan. After counselling she chooses to have medical treatment for the ectopic pregnancy.

    Which is the most appropriate treatment?

    A   Methotrexate 75 mg IM once

    B   Methotrexate 5 mg PO daily for 14 days

    C   Mifepristone 600 mg PO once

    D   Misoprostol 400 µg PO once

    E   No treatment

50. What is the greatest risk factor for placental abruption?

    A   Breech presentation

    B   Fibroid uterus

    C   Placental abruption in previous pregnancy

    D   Pre-eclampsia

    E   Previous caesarean section

51. Which of the following statements describes the action of calcitonin?

    A   It acts in the renal tubule to promote calcium reabsorption

    B   It acts in the renal tubule to reduce phosphate reabsorption

    C   It increases osteoclast activity

    D   It inhibits osteoblast activity

    E   It promotes vitamin D activation

52. Which of the following is an inhibitor of lactation?

    A   A fall in oestrogen levels

    B   Cabergoline therapy

    C   Infant suckling

    D   Prolactin

    E   Reduced progesterone levels after delivery

53. Which of the following ovarian tumours is responsible for the majority of ovarian malignancies?

    A   Brenner's tumour

    B   Dermoid cyst

    C   Ovarian fibroma

    D   Serous cystadenocarcinoma

    E   Sertoli–Leydig cell tumour

54. What percentage of teratomas of the ovary are bilateral?

    A   1%
    B   5%
    C   10%
    D   15%
    E   20%

55. Which of the following primary bone tumours is malignant in nature?

    A   Chondroma
    B   Haemangioma
    C   Fibroma
    D   Osteoid osteoma
    E   Osteosarcoma

56. Which of the following is the most common form of cervical cancer?

    A   Adenocarcinoma
    B   Adenosquamous carcinoma
    C   Clear cell carcinoma
    D   Squamous cell carcinoma
    E   Villoglandular adenocarcinoma

57. Which of the following cytological changes is characteristic of cervical intraepithelial neoplasia?

    A   Decreased nuclear/cytoplasmic ratio
    B   Decreased mitotic activity
    C   Increased meiotic activity
    D   Koilocytosis
    E   Mononuclear cells

58. A 72-year-old woman has a sudden onset loss of speech and hemiparesis. On arrival in hospital her symptoms and neurological examination is suggestive of a cerebrovascular incident. Subsequent imaging supports the diagnosis of an ischaemic stroke, affecting her left cerebral hemisphere.

Which of the following forms of tissue necrosis is associated with her loss of function?

    A   Caseous necrosis
    B   Coagulative necrosis
    C   Colliquative necrosis
    D   Fat necrosis
    E   Gangrenous necrosis

59. A 24-year-old primiparous woman is 10 weeks pregnant. She is known to have a form of thrombophilia, as do members of her immediate family. Her booking midwife refers her for obstetric-led care.

Which of the following is a congenital thrombophilia?

A   Antiphospholipid syndrome
B   Heparin induced thrombocytopaenia
C   Nephrotic syndrome
D   Paroxysmal nocturnal haemoglobinuria
E   Protein C deficiency

60. A 33-year-old nulliparous woman is referred to a recurrent miscarriage clinic by her general practitioner. She has had four consecutive first trimester miscarriages. She would like preconception advice and investigation.

Which of the following is an acquired thrombophilia?

A   Antiphospholipid syndrome
B   Antithrombin III deficiency
C   Dysfibrinogenemia
D   Factor V Leiden
E   Protein S deficiency

61. A computed tomography (CT) scan is arranged for a woman in pain post subtotal abdominal hysterectomy, to investigate the possibility of an intra-abdominal collection.

The unit for measurement for effective radiation dose is Sievert (Sv). What is the approximate effective radiation dose with a CT of the Abdomen and Pelvis?

A   0.1 mSV
B   1 mSV
C   10 mSV
D   100 mSV
E   1000 mSV

62. During electrosurgery, current modulation is important to achieve different tissue effects.

Which mode will provide a blend of 50% on and 50% off?

A   Continuous mode
B   Modulated Blend 1 mode
C   Modulated Blend 2 mode
D   Modulated Blend 3 mode
E   Coagulation mode

63. Radioisotopes are often used as sources of delivering radiotherapy. Isotopes of iodine can be used in the treatment of thyroid cancer. The symbol of a frequently used radioisotope is shown below:

^{131}I

What is number of neutrons in this isotope?

A   0

B 53
C 78
D 131
E 184

64. Which of the following is an acute side effect of radiotherapy?

   A Epithelial surface damage
   B Hair loss
   C Infertility
   D Lymphoedema
   E Tissue fibrosis

65. A 36-year-old woman who has had one previous vaginal delivery is seen in antenatal clinic at 36-weeks' gestation. She is keen to avoid further pregnancy in the next year or so, although she intends to have more children in the future. Having discussed the contraceptive options available to her she opts to have an intrauterine device (IUD) fitted after her baby is born?

   How soon after the delivery of her baby can this patient's IUD be inserted?

   A Immediately after delivery of the placenta
   B Two weeks postpartum
   C Four weeks postpartum
   D Six weeks postpartum
   E Six months postpartum

66. A 26-year-old woman attends the emergency department feeling unwell and complaining of lower abdominal pain. On examination she has a temperature of 39°C and a pulse rate of 110 beats per minute. She has lower abdominal tenderness with guarding and cervical excitation. A speculum examination reveals profuse discharge.

   What is the most immediate appropriate management?

   A Admit for intravenous antibiotics and supportive care
   B Book for a diagnostic laparoscopy
   C Organise a pelvic ultrasound scan
   D Refer for a surgical review
   E Refer to a sexual health clinic for screening and partner contact tracing

67. A 27-year-old female teacher, who is 14 weeks pregnant, presents to her general practitioner as she is concerned because one of her students was sent home today with chickenpox. Her varicella zoster virus IgG antibody is positive.

   What is the correct advice to give her?

   A Chickenpox is not contagious once the rash appears so she need not worry
   B She is immune to chickenpox and no further action needs to be taken
   C She should have be referred to fetal medicine unit for a scan to exclude abnormality

    D   She should not attend the hospital as she may infect other pregnant women

    E   She should receive varicella zoster immune globulin within the next 24 hours for it to be effective

68. A 28-year-old patient attends outpatient clinic with primary subfertility. Her partner's semen analysis and her hysterosalpingogram are normal. Her follicle-stimulating hormone is 2.3 IU/mL, luteinising hormone is 6.8 IU/mL and her day 21 progesterone is 19 ng/mL.

What is the most likely cause for her subfertility?

    A   Asherman's syndrome

    B   Endometriosis

    C   Hypogonadotrophic hypogonadism

    D   Premature menopause

    E   Polycystic ovarian syndrome

69. A fetal blood sample is performed on a primiparous 24-year-old woman at 7 cm dilatation due to a pathological cardiotocograph (CTG). The result shows a pH of 7.24.

Which is the most appropriate action based on this result?

    A   A repeat sample should be performed in 30 minutes

    B   It is a normal result and the patient should be reassured

    C   A repeat sample should be performed in 60 minutes

    D   Proceed straight to caesarean section

    E   The patient should be placed into left lateral position

70. An 18-year-old pregnant woman attends antenatal clinic at 32 weeks' gestation. Her urine sample reveals protein + and leucocytes +. She is asymptomatic of a urinary tract infection and is otherwise well.

What is the most appropriate action?

    A   Antibiotics and send urine for microscopy and culture

    B   Blood tests including a full blood count and renal function

    C   Renal ultrasound scan and antibiotics

    D   Routine urine dipstick at next appointment

    E   Send urine for microscopy and culture and treat if positive

71. A 22-year-old primiparous woman books her pregnancy at 11 weeks' gestation. Her booking blood tests reveal a haemoglobin level of 10.1 g/dL. Electrophoresis reveals haemoglobin karyotype HbAS.

What is the diagnosis?

    A   Beta-thalassaemia major

    B   Beta-thalassaemia trait

    C   Hereditary spherocytosis

    D   Sickle cell anaemia

    E   Sickle cell trait

72. A 32-year-old woman is being continuously monitored during labour using a cardiotocograph (CTG). She has had one previous caesarean section for breech presentation at term. She is currently 40 weeks' gestation and in spontaneous labour. The baseline of the CTG is 115 beats per minute.

Regarding CTG analysis, what is the accepted range for the baseline rate?

A   80–100 beats per minute
B   90–120 beats per minute
C   110–150 beats per minute
D   110–160 beats per minute
E   120–180 beats per minute

73. A 32-year-old multiparous pregnant woman attends the antenatal clinic for review at 28 weeks' gestation. She mentions that her 4-year-old daughter has chickenpox. She is unsure whether she has had chickenpox before. Serology results are as follows:

Varicella zoster virus IgM: negative
Varicella zoster virus IgG: positive

What do the serology results suggest regarding her immune status with respect to chickenpox?

A   Acute episode of shingles
B   Varicella zoster – chronic carrier
C   Varicella zoster – current acute infection
D   Varicella zoster – no acute infection, no previous exposure
E   Varicella zoster – previous exposure

74. A 40-year-old primiparous woman is admitted and investigated for raised blood pressure. Protein shows +++ on urine dipstick. A 24-hour urine collection is sent for protein calculation.

What level of urinary protein excretion in 24 hours indicates significant proteinuria?

A $>0.1\,g$
B $>0.2\,g$
C $>0.3\,g$
D $>0.4\,g$
E $>0.5\,g$

75. Haemolytic disease of the newborn (Rhesus incompatibility) occurs as a result of which of the following classes of hypersensitivity reaction?

A   IgE mediated
B   Immune complex mediated
C   Type I
D   Type II
E   Type IV

76. Which of the following gives the structure of the antibody IgG?

	Structure	Properties
A	Dimer	Main immunoglobulin found in secretions, e.g. saliva, and mucosal surfaces
B	Monomer	Antigen receptor on B cells
C	Monomer	Main mediator of allergic reaction
D	Monomer	Only immunoglobulin to cross the placenta
E	Pentamer	First immunoglobulin to be produced; expressed on surface of B cells

77. What is the common step to all complement activation pathways?

- **A** Activation of C1 to antibody-antigen complexes
- **B** Cleavage of C3 into C3a and C3b
- **C** Formation of the mannose-binding lectin complex
- **D** Formation of the IgG antibody-antigen complex
- **E** Formation of the IgM antibody-antigen complex

78. A 32-year-old woman presents to hospital 5 days post-emergency caesarean section, complaining of a painful scar. On examination, there is erythema at one of the scar edges and some purulent discharge. She is started on antibiotic treatment for a wound infection.

Which of the following local changes can be seen in this type of acute inflammatory process?

- **A** Fibroblast infiltration
- **B** Haemostasis
- **C** High concentration of monocytes
- **D** Decreased vascular permeability
- **E** Vasoconstriction

79. A 50-year-old woman has pelvic pain; she has had a coil in situ for the last 8 years. She has a pelvic mass; histological sampling of the mass at laparoscopy shows a suppurative and granulomatous inflammatory process with the presence of sulphur granules.

Which is the most likely causative agent?

- **A** *Actinomyces israelii*
- **B** *Chlamydia trachomatis*
- **C** *Gardnerella vaginalis*
- **D** *Neisseria gonorrhoeae*
- **E** *Neisseria meningitidis*

80. An 18-year-old woman presents to a sexual health clinic requesting a sexually transmitted infection screen; she is asymptomatic, however she is concerned as her new boyfriend is complaining of dysuria, penile discharge and scrotal pain.

What is the most likely cause of his symptoms?

A   *Actinomyces israelii*
B   *Candida albicans*
C   *Chlamydia trachomatis*
D   *Toxoplasma gondii*
E   *Treponema pallidum pallidum*

81. A 35-year-old man presents at a sexual health clinic with a new painless round lesion on his penis; he also has non-tender inguinal lymphadenopathy.

What is the most likely causative agent of his symptoms?

A   *Chlamydia trachomatis*
B   *Neisseria gonorrhoeae*
C   *Treponema pallidum carateum*
D   *Treponema pallidum pallidum*
E   *Treponema pallidum pertenue*

82. A 63-year-old man with an open fracture of the femur develops the rare complication of gas gangrene and requires leg amputation.

What is the most likely causative agent?

A   *Clostridium botulinum*
B   *Clostridium perfringens*
C   *Clostridium tetani*
D   *Escherichia coli*
E   *Klebsiella pneumonia*

83. A 28-year-old primiparous woman who is 16 weeks pregnant reports mild dysuria; otherwise she is well. Urine dipstick shows leucocytes ++ and is positive for nitrites. She is prescribed appropriate antibiotics.

What is the most likely causative organism of her urinary tract infection?

A   *Citrobacter freundii*
B   *Escherichia coli*
C   *Klebsiella pneumoniae*
D   *Proteus mirabilis*
E   *Staphylococcus saprophyticus*

84. Which of the following is the causative agent of Kaposi's sarcoma?

A   HIV
B   Human herpesvirus 4
C   Human herpesvirus 8
D   Human T-lymphotrophic virus 1
E   All of the above

85. A 32-year-old primiparous schoolteacher is 16 weeks pregnant. She is seen in the antenatal clinic, where she reports a maculopapular rash and coryzal symptoms.

The general practitioner has already sent serology and you review the result.

Rubella IgG: positive
Rubella IgM: negative
Parvovirus B19 IgG: negative
Parvovirus B19 IgM: positive

What is the most likely diagnosis?

A   Non-immunity to parvovirus B19
B   Non-immunity to rubella
C   Recent infection with rubella
D   Recent infection with parvovirus B19
E   None of the above

86. A 35-year-old multiparous woman has presented to labour ward in spontaneous labour. You see from her antenatal notes that she is HIV-positive. She is currently using highly active antiretroviral therapy and has a viral load of 43 copies/mL.

Which of the following is associated with increased risk of vertical transmission of HIV?

A   Co-existent Group B *Streptococcus* carriage
B   Chorioamnionitis
C   Paternal HIV-infection
D   Post-dates gestation
E   Vaginal examination during labour

87. Which type of uterine fibroid is found in the tissue layer adjacent to the endometrium?

A   Intramural
B   Intraserosal
C   Pedunculated subserosal
D   Submucosal
E   Subserosal

88. Sarcomas are the result of malignant transformation of which type of cell?

A   Blast
B   Epithelial
C   Hematopoietic
D   Mesenchyme
E   Pluripotent

89. Which of the following is a risk factor for osteoporosis?

A   Caffeine intake
B   Hyperparathyroidism
C   Late menarche
D   Nulliparity
E   Obesity

90. Which of the following statements correctly describes metaplastic change?

    A   Abnormal nuclear changes
    B   A decrease in the number of cells
    C   An increase in the number of cells
    D   An increase in cell size
    E   Transformation from one type of differentiated cell to another type of cell

91. In addition to mast cells, which of the following cells produces histamine?

    A   Basophils
    B   Erythrocytes
    C   Macrophages
    D   Monocytes
    E   Neutrophils

92. Within what timeframe from injury do macrophages replace neutrophils in cutaneous wound healing?

    A   1–2 hours
    B   6–12 hours
    C   18–24 hours
    D   48–92 hours
    E   7–10 days

93. A 40-year-old primiparous woman is admitted to the labour ward at 36 weeks' gestation with severe pre-eclampsia and presumed renal involvement. Her blood pressure on arrival is 184/95 mmHg. Her urine contains protein +++. Her serum creatinine is 92 μmol/L and serum urea 5.3 mg/dL.

Which of the following best describes the renal pathology of pre-eclampsia?

    A   Atheromatous plaques
    B   Glomerular capillary endotheliosis
    C   Glomerular hypertrophy
    D   Mesangial cell hypertrophy
    E   Tubular vacuolisation

94. A 45-year-old woman is seen in the gynaecology outpatient clinic with a history of severe menorrhagia. She has a body mass index of 42 kg/m². An endometrial biopsy is taken at hysteroscopy, which shows evidence of simple endometrial hyperplasia.

Which of the following describes the type of cellular change that occurs in hyperplasia?

    A   Increase in the number of cells
    B   Increase in the number of mitotic figures
    C   Increase in the number of nuclei in each cell
    D   Increase in the size of cells
    E   Increase in the thickness of the cell

95. A 30-year-old woman has an intrauterine death at 35 weeks' gestation. After delivery of the fetus, cabergoline is given to prevent lactation.

What is the main mechanism of action of cabergoline?

    A   Dopamine receptor D1 agonist
    B   Dopamine receptor D1 antagonist
    C   Dopamine receptor D2 agonist
    D   Dopamine receptor D2 antagonist
    E   Serotonin receptor agonist

96. A 33-year-old woman presents at 34 weeks' gestation with severe pre-eclampsia. Her blood pressure is 170/100 mmHg.

What is the first line oral agent to manage the hypertension?

    A   Labetolol
    B   Nifedipine
    C   Methyldopa
    D   Magnesium sulphate
    E   Hydralazine

97. A 30-year-old woman with severe pre-eclampsia has a post-partum haemorrhage following an instrumental delivery.

Which of the following uterotonics is contraindicated in pre-eclampsia?

    A   Carboprost
    B   Syntocinon IM
    C   Ergometrine
    D   Misoprostol
    E   Syntocinon IV

98. A 25-year-old woman has an intrauterine fetal death at 38 weeks' gestation. After appropriate counselling she consents for induction of labour. She is given mifepristone and admitted 24 hours later for misoprostol to induce labour.

To which class of drug does mifepristone belong?

    A   Anti-progesterone
    B   Anti-prostaglandin
    C   Ergot alkaloid
    D   GnRH analogue
    E   Prostaglandin

99. A 25-year-old woman is 6 weeks pregnant and presents with vaginal spotting, with no haemodynamic compromise. Following a pelvic ultrasound scan a left-sided ectopic pregnancy is confirmed. After counselling, she opts for medical management with methotrexate.

To which class of drug does methotrexate belong?

    A   Anti-progesterone

B Anti-prostaglandin
C Ergot alkaloid
D GnRH analogue
E Inhibits folic acid metabolism

100. A 32-year-old woman gave birth by caesarean section due to fetal distress at 41 weeks' gestation. She is now Para 4. The estimated blood loss was 1300 mL. Her booking BMI was 28 kg/m² with a weight of 70 kg.

What thromboprophylaxis is recommended in the postnatal period?

A No thromboprophylaxis required
B Inpatient low molecular weight heparin (LMWH) only
C 10 days LMWH
D 6 weeks LMWH
E 6 weeks Warfarin

Answers

1. B 1–20 MHz

Ultrasound is a non-ionising imaging modality that uses very high frequency sound waves. The frequencies typically used in modern ultrasonography range from 1–10 MHz, however ultrasonography can sometimes use frequencies of up to 20 MHz. An abdominal ultrasound typically uses wave frequencies of 2–3 MHz, whereas transvaginal ultrasound uses a higher frequency of around 5 MHz. In addition to producing images, ultrasound can be used to provide therapeutic interventions. For example, lithotripsy is a modality of treatment for renal stones using ultrasound technology. **Figure 16.1** shows an ultrasound image of a uterine fibroid.

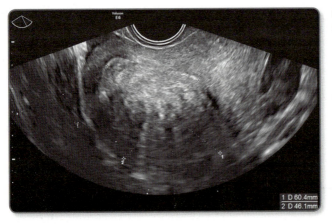

Figure 16.1 Ultrasound image showing uterine fibroid.

2. B 1 in 200

Women who have undergone delivery by previous caesarean section need adequate counselling early in the antenatal period in order to ensure that the subsequent delivery proceeds safely. Women who have had a previous uncomplicated lower segment caesarean section at term can usually be offered a vaginal birth after a caesarean (VBAC), providing there are no contraindications to a vaginal delivery. One specific risk that women should be counselled about is the risk of uterine rupture through the previous scar. This is frequently quoted as 1 in 200 and it should be explained to women that this is one of the reasons for continuous monitoring via cardiotocograph. The risk of hypoxic ischaemic encephalopathy (HIE) is 8 per 10 000 (0.08%) with a VBAC compared to <1 per 10000 (<0.1%) with planned elective repeat caesarean section

3. C 5–6 weeks

Evidence of fetal heart action depends on the mode of ultrasound and the gestation. Transvaginal ultrasound provides earlier visualisation of the fetal heart, which should be evident from 5–6 weeks' gestation. If trans-abdominal ultrasound is used, fetal heart action may not be seen until 6–7 weeks' gestation. Transvaginal ultrasound doesn't need the urinary bladder to be full, contrary to transabdominal ultrasound where an empty bladder leads to very poor visualisation of the pelvis.

4. C QRS complex

The electrocardiogram (ECG) pictorially represents electrical activity in the heart, with the resultant waveforms signifying both the location in the heart where the electrical activity is taking place and also the direction of electrical conduction. In the standard 12-lead ECG the P wave represents the passage of electricity from the sino-atrial node through the atria, causing atrial depolarisation. The PR interval represents the time it takes for the electrical signal to pass from the sino-atrial node, through the atria and then to the atrio-ventricular node ready to begin ventricular depolarisation. It is the QRS complex that represents the depolarisation of the ventricles. The T wave represents repolarisation of the ventricles, whereas the QT interval signifies the time taken for the sequential ventricular depolarisation, followed by repolarisation, to occur.

5. D Standard 2 weeks of antibiotic treatment

Women who have HIV and are diagnosed with pelvic inflammatory disease should be treated with the same antibiotic regimens as non-HIV positive women. They may present with more clinically severe symptoms but should respond just as well to treatment. Hospital admission should be considered based on individual clinical findings and is not mandatory. Women who are on antiretroviral drugs should be managed in conjunction with their HIV specialist doctor to prevent drug interactions.

6. D Referral to a genitourinary physician for treatment in line with her condition

If a woman presents with primary genital herpes during her pregnancy, she should be referred to a genitourinary unit. She is likely to need antivirals such as acyclovir in oral or intravenous form, depending on the severity of her symptoms.

As there is the risk of vertical transmission at delivery, any woman who presents towards the end of her pregnancy (within 6 weeks of likely delivery) needs investigation to establish whether there is primary or secondary infection. Type specific herpes simplex virus antibody testing differentiates between primary and secondary herpes. Detection of IgG antibodies matching those from genital swabs confirms secondary herpes.

Caesarean section is the recommended mode of delivery for women who have primary genital herpes confirmed within 6 weeks of their anticipated delivery date. Women with recurrent genital herpes infection should not routinely be offered a Caesarean section.

7. A Laparoscopy and dye test

Primary subfertility with painful periods for a long duration raises the suspicion of chronic conditions like endometriosis, fibroids and chronic pelvic inflammatory disease (PID). Ultrasound and clinical examination may help in diagnosis, but definitive diagnosis of endometriosis and adhesions can only be made effectively with laparoscopy. Performing a dye test also allows for the assessment of tubal patency.

8. D Intravenous access and resuscitation

This patient has had a placental abruption. The finding of a hard, tender abdomen is suggestive of a major abruption, which may have led to fetal demise. Not all women with placental abruption will present with revealed vaginal bleeding. Risk factors for placental abruption include previous abruption, advanced maternal age, pre-eclampsia, polyhydramnios, intrauterine infection, pregnancy following assisted reproduction, fetal growth restriction, drug use and smoking.

Maternal resuscitation and prompt multi-disciplinary care is paramount. Blood and clotting factors will need to be requested and transfused as necessary. Ultrasound should be carried out to establish if there has been intrauterine death. If there is fetal demise, a vaginal delivery is generally aimed for. Women who have abruption in one pregnancy are more likely to have a recurrence in future pregnancies.

9. A Call for immediate help

When faced with any collapsed patient, you must always ask for help immediately.

The patient should be actively resuscitated and treatment for a postpartum haemorrhage (PPH) initiated. The causes of PPH are often classified as the four Ts; Tone, Trauma, Tissue and Thrombin (**Table 16.1**).

Table 16.1 Causes of postpartum haemorrhage	
Causes of postpartum haemorrhage	**Risk factors**
Tone	Placenta praevia
	Grand multiparity
	Multiple pregnancy
	Obesity
	Increasing age
	History of postpartum haemorrhage
Thrombin	Pre-eclampsia
	Placental abruption
	Pyrexia in labour
Tissue	Retained placenta
Trauma	Caesarean section
	Operative vaginal delivery
	Big baby

10. D Perform a urine dipstick to assess for proteinuria

Pregnant women should have their urine checked for protein at every antenatal visit.
If protein is detected, a urine tract infection and pre-eclampsia should be excluded.
Ankle oedema is very common in pregnancy, and is in itself not a worrying sign.
A diagnosis of hypertension cannot be made on a single blood pressure reading.
Recognised risk factors for pre-eclampsia in pregnancy are advanced maternal age,
obesity, multiple pregnancy, chronic hypertension and pre-existing diabetes. See
Table 16.2 for classification of hypertension in pregnancy.

Table 16.2 Classification of hypertension in pregnancy	
Classification of hypertension in pregnancy	**Blood pressure ranges (systolic/diastolic)**
Mild	140/90–149/99 mmHg
Moderate	150/100–159/109 mmHg
Severe	≥160/110 mmHg

11. C Intravenous antibiotics followed by an ERPC

Retained products of conception may persist after a spontaneous miscarriage and
occasionally after an evacuation of the retained products of conception (ERPC).
In this case there is evidence of infection, and prior to any surgical intervention it
would be appropriate to administer intravenous antibiotics to reduce the chance of
uterine perforation.

12. E Premature ovarian failure

Premature ovarian failure, or premature menopause, is defined as the onset of menopause before the age of 40 years. The most common presentation is amenorrhoea or oligomenorrhoea and there may be co-existing medical conditions. Possible causes and the corresponding investigations and treatments are listed in **Table 16.3**.

Table 16.3 Causes of premature ovarian failure with investigation and treatment options

Cause	Investigations	Treatment
Primary: genetic, autoimmune disease, Turner's syndrome, enzyme deficiencies	Follicle-stimulating hormone level is high, usually above >30 IU/L	Management of infertility if conception is desired
Secondary: chemotherapy, infection, hysterectomy +/– oophorectomy	Levels of oestradiol, luteinising hormone and progesterone are of limited value	Women usually need oestrogen replacement until the age of approximately 52 years

13. B Anticardiolipin antibodies

Thrombophilia may be acquired or inherited, and results in a high-risk of thromboembolic events. Thrombophilia in pregnancy results in an even higher risk. Inherited thrombophilias include protein C and S deficiency, antithrombin III deficiency and activated protein C resistance (Factor V Leiden). Activated protein C resistance is autosomal dominant and in individuals heterozygous for the condition, there is up to a 10 times greater lifetime risk of thrombosis.

Antiphospholipid syndrome is an acquired thrombophilia and is found in approximately 15% of women presenting with recurrent miscarriage. Antiphospholipid syndrome can be diagnosed when there are anticardiolipin antibodies or lupus anticoagulant with three or more consecutive miscarriages before 10 weeks with or without thrombosis. Some of these conditions may not be revealed until a precipitating event occurs, such as pregnancy. All women with thrombophilia are classed as high-risk.

14. C Sarcoidosis

Sarcoidosis is a granulomatous disease that affects many body systems. The granulomata are non-caseating, unlike in tuberculosis. It mainly affects adults aged 20–40 years, however prevalence during pregnancy is uncommon, affecting only 0.05% of all pregnancies. It is often asymptomatic and may be discovered incidentally. Symptoms of pulmonary disease include a dry cough, shortness of breath and chest pain. Extrapulmonary signs include erythema nodosum, uveitis, fever and hypercalcaemia. Erythema nodosum usually manifests as painful, red lesions on the arms and legs and may occur spontaneously in pregnancy without any underlying pathology. The most common feature on a chest X-ray is bilateral hilar lymphadenopathy, but there may also be evidence of fibrosis. Serum levels of serum angiotensin-converting enzyme may be altered in pregnancy and therefore are not a useful marker of disease. Pregnancy can often lead to an improvement in the disease, which is thought to occur as a result of increased levels of cortisol.

15. A 5–25 beats per minute

Beat-to-beat variability is normal and should be between 5 and 25 beats per minute. Variability increases as the gestational age increases. Sleep patterns, movement and periods of accelerations and decelerations will affect the variability in heart rate. It may be normal for the fetus to have a sleep pattern for up to 90 minutes; however, this only becomes evident on a cardiotocography trace after 28 weeks' gestation.

16. B Chronic infection

Hepatitis B serology screening forms part of the standard booking blood tests. During an acute infection, hepatitis B surface antigen is found in the serum and is positive. Presence of hepatitis B core antibody indicates previous infection and would usually be detected in the blood 6 weeks after the initial infection. The surface antigen disappears if the infection becomes inactive and the surface antibody is then formed. Chronic infection is indicated in this case, as the patient is positive for hepatitis surface antigen and core antibody. If the acute infection is not cleared from the bloodstream, then there is a risk of developing liver cirrhosis in the future. Hepatitis infection during pregnancy poses a risk of vertical transmission. All babies born to mothers with hepatitis B infection are vaccinated at birth, with the addition of immunoglobulin if the mother is highly infectious.

17. E 65 pmol/L

Hirsutism is characterised by coarse hairs with a male-like distribution. It may affect up to 15% of women. Polycystic ovary syndrome (PCOS) is the most common cause of hirsutism. This patient's hormone profile is suggestive of PCOS. Her anti-Müllerian hormone level is raised, both of which are consistent with this diagnosis.

It can be difficult to make a diagnosis of PCOS and therefore the Rotterdam Criteria are used once other causes have been excluded. The Rotterdam Criteria make a diagnosis on the basis of the presence at least two out of three of features of (1) polycystic ovaries on ultrasound scan, (2) oligo/anovulation and (3) hyperandrogenism (clinical or biochemical). On presentation this patient meets two of the criteria.

Hirsutism is distressing to many women. A standardised scoring system such as Ferriman–Gallwey score may be useful to evaluate efficacy of treatment, which may be cosmetic, medical or a combination of both. Medical treatment may include a combination of oestrogen and antiandrogen, cyproterone acetate. Weight reduction of 5–10% can induce an improvement in hirsutism by 40–55% within 6 months of weight loss. In obese women with PCOS, a weight loss programme should be the first line of intervention.

18. D 5000 IU/L

In early pregnancy, a transvaginal ultrasound combined with serum human chorionic gonadotropin (hCG) has a very high positive predictive for diagnosing an ectopic pregnancy. A singleton intrauterine pregnancy should be visible with hCG from 1000–2400 IU/L. Multiple pregnancies may be visible with higher hCG values.

The diagnosis of ectopic pregnancy should be based on the identification of an extra-uterine sac and indirect signs such as a complex adnexal mass or free fluid. Women with a pregnancy of unknown location could have an ectopic pregnancy until the location is determined. In a woman with a pregnancy of unknown location, clinical symptoms are more important than serum hCG results.

19. D Streptococcal nephritis

Streptococcal nephritis is an example of type III reaction where there is immune complex deposition. In Goodpasture's syndrome type II hypersensitivity reactions occur.

Blood transfusion reactions are another example of a form of type II hypersensitivity. In this reaction antibodies are directed against antigen on the individual's cells. Type I reactions are caused by immediate activation of IgE antibody and can also be described as anaphylactic hypersensitivity. Type IV reactions are associated with activation of T-lymphocytes. Type IV hypersensitivity reactions occur in conditions such as tuberculosis, rheumatoid arthritis and multiple sclerosis (**Table 16.4**).

Table 16.4 Hypersensitivity reactions		
Timing	**Type**	**Mechanism**
Immediate	I	IgE antibodies
5–8 hours	II	Antibody and complement
2–8 hours	III	Immune complex
> 24 hours	IV	T-cell mediated
> 12 hours	V	Antibody mediated

20. D IgG

Immunoglobin (IgG) is the most plentiful of the immunoglobulin isotopes and is fundamental to the secondary immune response. It is also the only form of antibody that is able to cross the placenta and by doing so confers the growing fetus with passive immunity. Maternal IgA is found in large quantities in breast milk and therefore confers passive immunity to the newborn. The immune system of the fetus starts to develop early on in the first trimester and includes the production of complement and the antibody IgM. IgA has been detected in fetal serum during the third trimester.

21. C Opsonisation

The complement system forms part of both the innate and acquired immune systems. The complement proteins produced by the liver are activated in the form of a cascade via three different pathways (classical, alternative and lectin). The different products of each stage of the complement cascade have different roles. Opsonisation is one of the major functions of the complement system. Complement proteins cover the surfaces of pathogens, such as bacteria, which then attract cells such as macrophages, which phagocytose the pathogen. The complement protein C3b is the main protein involved in opsonisation. Other functions of the complement system include cell lysis, chemotaxis, increasing vascular permeability by stimulating histamine release and activation of the lipoxygenase pathway.

22. C *Gardnerella vaginalis*

Bacterial vaginosis (BV) is caused by overgrowth of the anaerobic bacterium *Gardnerella vaginalis* together with other bacteria such as *Prevotella* species, *Mobiluncus* species and *Mycoplasma hominis*. Amsel's criteria can be used to aid diagnosis when three of the following are present: (1) thin white homogenous discharge, (2) clue cells on microscopy, (3) pH of vaginal secretions > 4.5 and (4) fishy odour on adding alkali (the whiff test). Women may be asymptomatic or may notice increased foul-smelling vaginal discharge. Although not a sexually transmitted infection, there is a higher prevalence of BV in sexually active women. Treatment with antibiotic therapy such as metronidazole may provide relief, although it may self-resolve.

23. D *Treponema pallidum pertenue*

Human syphilis, yaws, pinta and bejel are all caused by different sub-species of the Gram-negative spirochaeta *Treponema pallidum*. Yaws is caused by *Treponema pallidum pertenue* and is a disease found in tropical areas of the world, where it manifests as an infection of skin, bones and joints. It may form infective cutaneous lesions and can be transmitted by skin to skin contact. Bejel is caused by *Treponema endemicum*, pinta by *Treponema carateum* and finally syphilis by *Treponema pallidum*. It is important to remember that infection with the non-venereal forms of *Treponema* will also cause a positive result on tests for syphilis, such as the fluorescent treponemal antibody–absorption (FTA–abs) test.

24. A dsDNA

Cytomegalovirus, also known as human herpesvirus 5, belongs to the herpes family of viruses and its genome consists of double-stranded DNA. The majority of adults will have been exposed to the virus and are seropositive if tested. Concern regarding the timing of exposure occurs during pregnancy, as fetal infection may be associated with an array of defects including microcephaly, hepatitis, cerebral palsy and sensorineural hearing loss. The answer stems given for this question derive from the Baltimore classification system. The system classifies viruses according to their genome, i.e. whether their nucleic acid is RNA or DNA, whether they are double-stranded (ds) or single-stranded (ss), their sense (+ or –) and whether their replication uses reverse transcriptase (RT).

25. D *Staphylococcus aureus*

Surgical wound infection is a common postoperative complication and standard policies are in place to try and minimise them. Examples of attempts to minimise wound infections include stringent hand hygiene, aseptic technique and in certain situations prophylactic antibiotics given at the time of procedure. Organisms enter the area of the wound from normal skin commensals, droplet spread and, specific to obstetrics and gynaecology, from the perineum or perianal region. Common pathogens implicated in wound infections are Gram-positive cocci, such as *Staphylococcus aureus*, which causes up to 20% of wound infections. Other common causes of infection include *Staphylococcus pyogenes* and *Escherichia coli*. Management would include appropriate resuscitative treatment including intravenous fluids, oxygen and prompt broad-spectrum antibiotics. Blood culture and a wound swab should also be taken prior to antibiotics.

26. E Underlying medical disorder

All of the above are potential operative risk factors. In this case, we know that there were no intraoperative complications and therefore the length of operation is unlikely to be a cause. Sterility of the instruments should be confirmed prior to operation and there should be no foreign material present after the operation.

Factors generally associated with an increased risk of wound infection are as follows.

Operative factors:

- Length of operation
- Ventilation of theatre
- Sterility of instruments
- Contaminated or dirty surgery
- Foreign material at operation site

Preoperative skin preparation patient factors:

- Age
- Body mass index
- Smoker
- Diabetes mellitus
- Impaired immunity

27. E Peptidoglycan

Gram-staining detects the presence of peptidoglycan in bacterial cell walls. The Gram stain is therefore used to differentiate between Gram-positive and Gram-negative bacteria and it is the composition of the cell wall that gives them these properties. Gram-positive bacteria have a thicker peptidoglycan layer than Gram-negative bacteria. Gram-positive bacteria stain blue/black; gram-negative stain pink/red. The bacterial cell wall is made up of N-acetyl glucosamine and N-acetyl muramic acid linked to peptidoglycan. It is this lipid, sugar and polypeptide structure which is responsible for maintaining the rigidity of the cell wall. The presence of a slimy glycocalyx on the surface of the bacteria is protective against destruction, e.g. by antimicrobials. Mycolic acid is found in high concentrations in the cell walls of organisms that are classified as 'acid-fast', such as *Mycoplasma*.

28. D Smoking

An ectopic pregnancy occurs when the embryo implants outside the uterine cavity. The most common site for an ectopic pregnancy is within the fallopian tubes; however, they may also occur on the ovaries, the cornua of the uterus, the cervix and rarely the abdominal cavity. Smoking is known to have an association with ectopic pregnancy, however obesity is not a recognised risk factor.

Any form of previous pelvic surgery raises the risk of a subsequent ectopic pregnancy, e.g. appendicectomy, due to the occurrence of adhesions. Other risk factors include pelvic inflammatory disease (genital infection), previous ectopic pregnancy, tubal surgery, endometriosis, use of the coil and usage of the progesterone-only contraceptive pill.

29. E Increased endothelial permeability

Acute inflammation describes the initial changes in the process of inflammation, which are designed to neutralise or eliminate the cause of injury. Within the vasculature there is vasodilatation secondary to the action of histamine and nitric oxide and increased capillary permeability. Marginalisation of leucocytes occurs in the capillaries and is enhanced by the action of adhesion molecules. The rouleau effect may be seen as a result of erythrocytes collecting centrally. The usual axial blood flow is slowed with the subsequent development of stasis. Angiogenesis and fibrosis occur as part of chronic inflammation.

30. C Testicles

Choriocarcinoma is classified as both a form of gestational trophoblastic disease and also as a form of primary germ cell tumour. Rarely choriocarcinoma can be found as a germ cell tumour in the testicles and in the ovaries. When present in the testes choriocarcinoma is classified as a non-seminomatous germ cell tumour and is known to be the most aggressive and rapidly metastasising form of this type of tumour. More commonly, choriocarcinoma is described as a malignancy of trophoblastic cells and usually occurs following the development of a partial or complete molar pregnancy, although it can occur after normal pregnancy, ectopic pregnancy or following termination of pregnancy. This form of tumour macroscopically has a fleshy appearance, whereas microscopically there is an abundance of cytotrophoblasts and syncytiotrophoblasts with an absence of chorionic villi.

31. E Villous hypovascularity with evidence of infarction

Pre-eclampsia is a multisystem disorder associated with abnormal placentation. Its sequelae occur as a consequence of widespread endothelial dysfunction, increased vascular permeability and vasoconstriction. In pregnancies affected by pre-eclampsia the placenta is found to have a series of histological changes including placental infarcts, increased syncytial knots and villous hypovascularity. Retroplacental haematomas are also more common. These changes reflect earlier placental implantation which is inadequate to stand up to the demands of the growing fetus. The histological appearance of a mass of small capillaries and non-specific trophoblast hyperplasia is associated with choriocarcinoma, not pre-eclampsia.

32. C Hyperchromatism

The histological term dysplasia is used to describe abnormal changes, both architectural and cytological, in the development of a cell type.

Dysplasia is characterised by the following:

- Anisocytosis: cells of varying size
- Hyperchromatism: excessive pigmentation due to abnormal chromatin
- Poikilocytosis: abnormally shaped cells
- Presence of mitotic figures: indicative of high cell turnover
- Loss of cell orientation

Dysplasia typically occurs in response to an environmental stimulus, e.g. the dysplastic changes seen in Barrett's oesophagus occur in response to chronic exposure to stomach acid. These changes may be an indicator of malignant potential, but they may be reversible. The cervical intraepithelial neoplasia (CIN) grading system refers to the severity of dysplastic changes in the cervix, where CIN I refers to mild dysplasia, CIN II to moderate dysplasia and CIN III severe dysplasia.

33. E Pregnancy-induced idiopathic thrombocytopaenic purpura

In haemolytic anaemia there is premature destruction of red cells, together with the reduced lifespan of circulating red cells. In pregnancy, haemolysis may be seen in HELLP syndrome, and haemolytic uraemic syndrome (HUS).

Chronic idiopathic thrombocytopaenic purpura (ITP) is a platelet disorder, not a haemolytic disorder. It caused by the development of IgG autoantibodies to platelets. It may be secondary to a variety of conditions such as systemic lupus erythematosus (SLE) and HIV. The condition manifests with peripheral thrombocytopaenia, however examination of the bone marrow may reveal the presence of megakaryocytes.

Primary ITP is a diagnosis of exclusion and can only be made after secondary causes have been excluded. Treatment is supportive and may include the administration of corticosteroids.

Thrombotic thrombocytopaenic purpura (TTP) shares similarities with HUS, and in both conditions there is microvascular platelet aggregation. In HUS there is predominantly renal involvement. Although HUS in pregnancy is rare, it is associated with significant perinatal or maternal morbidity and mortality. Polymorphic eruption of pregnancy (PEP) is an itchy erythematous rash that has no known cause, although it usually occurs during a first pregnancy. The distinguishing feature is sparing of the umbilical region and both PEP and gestational diabetes are not associated with microangiopathic haemolytic anaemia.

34. E White cell count: $< 4 \times 10^9$ cells/L

Systemic inflammatory response syndrome (SIRS) refers to the multisystem response seen in adults following a non-specific insult. It can be caused by infection but may also be a response to causes such as trauma, burns, pancreatitis, haemorrhage or inflammation. SIRS can be diagnosed when there are two of the following:

- Heart rate > 90 beats per minute
- Temperature $> 38°C$ or $< 36°C$
- Respiratory rate of > 20 breaths per minute or a $P_{CO_2} < 4.3$ kPa (32 mmHg)
- White cell count $< 4 \times 10^9$ cells/L or $> 12 \times 10^9$ cells/L

SIRS should not be confused with sepsis, a term which should only be used when there is SIRS alongside sepsis. The Sepsis Six describes six key therapies which, when instigated rapidly, reduce the mortality and morbidity associated with sepsis. These therapies are giving high flow oxygen, taking blood cultures, starting intravenous antibiotics, giving intravenous fluid, checking the serum lactate and monitoring the hourly urine output. Additional management may include the administration of corticosteroids and inotropes. Untreated SIRS may result in end-organ damage and multi-organ failure and, in severe cases, may be fatal.

35. E Thyroid-stimulating hormone

The pituitary gland sits in a bony fossa at the base of the cranium. The adenohypophysis (also known as the anterior pituitary) is derived from oral ectoderm. The adenohypophysis can be further divided into the pars distalis, the pars intermedia and the pars tuberalis. The neurohypophysis (also known as the posterior pituitary) is derived from neural ectoderm and is in fact an extension of the hypothalamus.

Histological staining identifies three types of cells in the adenohypophysis: acidophils, basophils and chromophobes. Acidophils produce both growth hormone and prolactin. Basophils produce thyroid-stimulating hormone, adrenocorticotrophic hormone, follicle-stimulating hormone and luteinising hormone. The neurohypophysis produces oxytocin and antidiuretic hormone, also known as vasopressin.

36. C Prolactin-secreting adenoma

The pituitary gland is composed of a single anterior lobe and a posterior lobe, with the anterior lobe forming the majority of the gland. Prolactin-secreting adenomas, known as prolactinomas, are the commonest form of pituitary adenomas, which are the most common form of pituitary tumours. The most common site of a pituitary adenoma is the anterior lobe. Only one-third of adenomas infiltrate the brain. These tumours may be functional or non-functional and are typically found in adults of 30–60 years of age. Affected individuals may present with subfertility, amenorrhoea and galactorrhoea.

37. A Erythroplakia

Premalignant diseases are conditions that, if untreated, have a high likelihood of becoming malignant. Erythroplakia (and leukoplakia) are both precancerous conditions of the oropharynx. Other examples of premalignant conditions include Crohn's disease, ulcerative colitis and Barrett's oesophagus where there is chronic inflammation leading to increased risk of bowel and oesophageal cancers respectively. Actinic keratosis, if left untreated, may develop into squamous cell carcinoma. Cervical intraepithelial neoplasia has the potential to change into cervical cancer if not monitored and appropriately treated. Lichen sclerosus is not a premalignant condition, however it thought around 5% of women with the condition go on to develop vulval cancer. Neither lichen planus nor herpes simplex infection are associated with the subsequent development of malignant conditions.

38. C Early age of first sexual intercourse

The main risk factors for the development of cervical cancer include: early age for first sexual intercourse, overall number of sexual partners, smoking and use of the oral contraceptive. The latter is indirectly associated with cervical cancer as oral contraceptive pills may increase the susceptibility to HPV infection. Unsurprisingly woman who are immune-compromised, i.e. have HIV/AIDS or are on immunosuppressant drugs following an organ transplant, are more likely to develop cervical cancer. Cervical cancer is more common in women in deprived areas and therefore in those women with a lower socioeconomic status. Having a male partner who has been circumcised is associated with a lower risk for the development of cervical cancer. Early menarche is not a risk factor for cervical cancer.

39. D Obesity

The incidence of endometrial cancer in United Kingdom is around 20 per 100,000 women, the majority of which are postmenopausal. The combined oral contraceptive, especially in users of more than 10 years, halves the risk of this form of cancer. Endometrial hyperplasia is recognised as being a premalignant condition. Simple hyperplasia is likely to be treated with progesterone. Atypical hyperplasia on the other hand may indicate that cancer is already present on other parts of the uterus and, if not, will lead to endometrial cancer in 30% of cases. Invasion of endometrial cancer is local, through the myometrium and into the peritoneal cavity. An MRI is performed to assess the extent of myometrial invasion and stage the disease. Stage 1a and 1b disease are treated by performing a total abdominal hysterectomy (TAH) and bilateral oophorectomy (BSO). Stage 1c and 2a disease are treated by TAH and BSO, followed by radiotherapy. Risk factors for the disease are related to high levels of oestrogen (i.e. obesity) or many menses, i.e. nulliparous women and those of who have had a late menopause.

40. D HPV 16

Human papilloma virus (HPV) is a double-stranded DNA virus. There are many subtypes of the virus, 30 of which are present in the human genital tract. Most lead to focal epithelial proliferation. High-risk virus types commonly detected in women with CIN II and CIN III are HPV16, HPV18 and HPV31. However, the prevalence of HPV in sexually active women under 30 years old is as high as 40%, but most will clear it within 6–8 months. Being older and smoking decreases the chance of the virus being cleared. HPV2 and 63 are associated with the presence of common warts. HPV6 and 11 are commonly associated with anogenital warts.

41. D µ

There are three main opioid receptors: µ, δ and κ. It is now widely accepted that most of the analgesic effects of opioids are achieved through the µ receptor. All opioid receptors are G-protein coupled receptors and act through the inhibition of adenylate cyclase. Action at these receptors also leads to opening of potassium channels causing hyperpolarisation. There is also inhibition of release of neurotransmitter via inhibition of calcium release at the calcium channels. Other effects of opioids include dysphoria (κ receptor), reduced gastrointestinal motility (all receptors), respiratory depression (µ and δ receptors) and physical dependence (µ and κ receptors).

42. E Warfarin

Warfarin, a coumarin, is a teratogen and should be avoided during pregnancy. Alternative therapy with a low-molecular weight heparin is more appropriate in women who require anticoagulation during pregnancy. More teratogenic effects occur if warfarin is given during the first trimester and can lead to fetal warfarin syndrome. Warfarin given in the second and third trimesters is thought to be associated with a lower level of birth defects. Fetal warfarin syndrome, or embryopathy, includes low birth weight, nasal hypoplasia and chondrodysplasia punctata. It can also lead to more global central nervous system abnormalities such as learning difficulties and neurodevelopmental delay.

43. E Inhibits enzymic reduction of vitamin K

Warfarin is an oral anticoagulant and inhibits the vitamin K dependent synthesis of various clotting factors (II, VII, IX and X). It reduces the post-translational gamma carboxylation of glutamic acid in clotting factors II, VII, IX and X and this is achieved via enzymic reduction of vitamin K. As the process of this enzymic reduction is competitive with vitamin K, ingestion of vitamin K will affect the efficacy of the drug. The onset of action of warfarin is delayed until the clotting factors have been eliminated from the blood.

Heparin and low-molecular weight heparin (LMWH) act in a different way. They activate antithrombin III which in turn inhibits thrombin. LMWHs increase the action of antithrombin III on factor Xa, but do not change the effect on thrombin. Heparin is safe to use during pregnancy.

44. E Thiopental

To reduce the risk of gastric aspiration, rapid sequence induction with cricoid pressure is used. To minimize the placental transfer of anaesthetic agent to the fetus, catheterisation, cleaning and draping should be performed prior to administration of anaesthetic in order that the surgeon can begin the procedure immediately.

Intravenous anaesthetic agents:

- Thiopental: barbiturate, very high lipid solubility
- Etomidate: involuntary movements during induction
- Propofol: rapidly metabolised and recovery with no hangover, used especially for day-case surgery
- Ketamine: causes profound analgesia, blocks NMDA receptor
- Midazolam: benzodiazepine, used for preoperative sedation

45. B Progesterone-only subdermal implant

Patients are potentially fertile 3 weeks postpartum. Women may rely on lactation amenorrhoea for contraception as long as they are exclusively breastfeeding, less than 6 months post partum and the baby is not receiving supplementary feeding.

There are several options for postpartum women, however, this was a teenage pregnancy for someone with a hectic lifestyle, so reliable contraception must be advised. As she is breastfeeding, the combined oral contraceptive (COC) pill is contraindicated. As the pregnancy was unplanned, condoms may not be reliable enough. The progesterone-only subdermal implant is ideal as it can be inserted before discharge, is highly reliable and remains effective for 3 years.

46. E Oxytetracycline

Tetracyclines, such as doxycycline and oxytetracycline, are broad-spectrum bacteriostatic antibiotics giving them a wide variety of uses, including the treatment of acne. They are known to chelate calcium leading to tetracycline deposition in growing teeth and bone. Given in the second and third trimester of pregnancy may cause maternal hepatotoxicity and fetal teeth discolouration in addition to skeletal deformities. These effects can also theoretically occur with breastfeeding, although it has been speculated that the calcium in milk may help prevent teeth discolouration. Because of these risks, all tetracyclines should be avoided in pregnant women, those breastfeeding and in children under the age of 12 years.

47. E Ramipril

Ramipril is an angiotensin-converting enzyme (ACE) inhibitor and is used for the treatment of conditions such as hypertension and heart failure. It acts on the renin–angiotensin–aldosterone system, preventing the conversion of angiotensin I to angiotensin II and therefore reducing arterial pressure and cardiac load. Unfortunately the use of ACE inhibitors in pregnancy, particularly in the first trimester, is associated with problems such as fetal skull defects, cardiovascular malformation, fetal renal problems and oligohydramnios. Alternative treatments for hypertension in pregnancy include labetalol, a first line treatment choice, and nifedipine and methyldopa as a second-line therapy.

48. E Sodium valproate

All of the antiepileptic drugs (AEDs) are associated with an increased incidence of teratogenesis, which increases with the number of agents used. Sodium valproate, as a single agent, is associated with the greatest incidence of fetal malformation in comparison to other AEDs and is associated with abnormalities such as neural tube defects, cardiac defects, fetal growth restriction and craniofacial defects. Current NICE guidance recommends that sodium valproate should be avoided in pregnant women and cites data from the UK Epilepsy and Pregnancy Register from 2002. This found a 7.2% incidence of teratogenesis in pregnancies when the woman used sodium valproate, in comparison with incidences of 3% for lamotrigine and 2.3% for carbamazepine. There is limited data regarding the teratogenic risks of levetiracetam in pregnancy, however current evidence suggests this is less than the older antiepileptic drugs. Counselling of pregnant women with epilepsy is essential and should always include a discussion regarding the risks to both the mother and fetus if AEDs are discontinued.

49. A Methotrexate 75 mg IM once

The administration of methotrexate intramuscularly may be a suitable treatment for ectopic pregnancy in certain circumstances. Methotrexate is an antimetabolite, which inhibits folate reductase. Current RCOG guidance advises that the administering a single 75 mg intramuscular injection of methotrexate is a suitable treatment for ectopic pregnancy in cases where β-human chorionic gonadotropin (β-hCG) is < 3000 IU/mL. Mifepristone and misoprostol both have a role in termination of pregnancy and the medical management of miscarriage but are not suitable for the management of tubal ectopic pregnancy.

Royal College of Obstetricians & Gynaecologists. The Management of Tubal Pregnancy. Green-top Guideline 21. London: RCOG, 2004.

50. C Placental abruption in previous pregnancy

Placental abruption is where the placenta separates from the uterus prior to the delivery of the fetus. It is one of the most common causes of antepartum haemorrhage (bleeding from the vagina or genital tract after 24 weeks of pregnancy). There are several known risk factors for placental abruption, including pre-eclampsia, polyhydramnios, advanced maternal age and smoking. The greatest risk factor for placental abruption is an abruption in a previous pregnancy. Abruption complicates up to 25% of pregnancies where abruption has occurred in two previous pregnancies. Prevention of abruption is via the limitation of risk factors. In women who have had a pregnancy complicated by previous abruption, there may be an indication for antithrombotic therapy.

51. B It acts in the renal tubule to reduce phosphate reabsorption

Calcitonin is an amino acid that is synthesised by the parafollicular cells of the thyroid gland. Parafollicular cells are neuroendocrine in origin and are derived from the neural crest. These neuroendocrine cells make up only 0.2% of the total thyroid gland cells. Circulating levels of calcium regulate calcitonin. When there are high levels of calcium, the level of calcitonin increases and vice versa. The primary organ of action is in the bone where it reduces the activity of osteoclasts. In the renal tubules, calcitonin acts to reduce the reabsorption of phosphate and calcium.

52. B Cabergoline therapy

Prolactin is produced from the anterior pituitary gland. Its production and release is increased by thyrotrophin-releasing hormone and inhibited by dopamine. Cabergoline is a dopamine antagonist and is used to suppress lactation postpartum in cases of mothers who have suffered a stillbirth, have HIV or simply do not wish to breastfeed.

High levels of oestrogen and progesterone during pregnancy inhibit lactation, but a drop in the level of these hormones after delivery and suckling lead to on-going production of prolactin.

53. D Serous cystadenocarcinoma

Ovarian cancer is the most common gynaecological malignancy and over 50% of cases present in women aged 45–65 years. They are classified into different groups according to their cell type: epithelial, sex cord stromal or germ cell. They may be benign, borderline or malignant. The most common ovarian cancers are serous cystadenocarcinomas; these malignant tumours account for around 75% of primary ovarian cancers.

Serous cystadenoma is the most common benign epithelial tumour. They are bilateral in 10% of cases. Mucinous cystadenoma are typically unilateral and larger in comparison to serous cystadenoma. The majority of Brenner tumours are benign with 10–15% being bilateral. They are generally small in size. Some Brenner tumours secrete oestrogen so may cause irregular vaginal bleeding.

Most common ovarian tumours in young women are benign germ cell tumours. They contain elements of all three layers of embryonic tissue.

54. C 10%

Teratomas are germ cell tumours of the ovary. They are typically benign, occurring in women under the age of 30 years. Only 10% of teratomas are bilateral. They rarely rupture and in most cases patients are asymptomatic, however up to 10% result in torsion and patients may present with an acute abdomen. They are mostly unilocular and thin-walled. The vast majority of ovarian teratomas are mature and cystic and are known as dermoid cysts. They usually measure < 20 cm.

55. E Osteosarcoma

Osteosarcomas are the most common malignant primary bone tumour and are a form of mesenchymal tumour. Most commonly they are found at the metaphysis of long bones. Chondromas are benign tumours of hyaline cartilage. Haemangiomas are not a type of bone tumour and actually describe benign tumours characterised by blood vessels filled with blood. They are typically seen in infancy and often spontaneously resolve. Fibromas are benign tumours of fibrous connective tissue. Osteoid osteomas are small benign bone tumours that most commonly arise in young adults.

56. D Squamous cell carcinoma

Around 80% of cervical cancers are squamous cell carcinomas. Adenocarcinomas are thought to be increasing in incidence and are present in around 10% of cases. Clear cell carcinoma of the cervix occurs in 1% of cases. This form of cervical cancer is historically associated with in utero exposure to diethylstilbestrol. Glassy cell carcinomas of the cervix are very rare and associated with < 1% of cases and typically present with vaginal bleeding in the absence of an abnormal smear. Other rare forms of cervical cancer include neuroendocrine tumours. By far the majority of cervical cancers are caused by HPV infection. Unfortunately some cervical tumour types are less effectively detected by national screening programmes and typically present at a more advanced stage, e.g. adenocarcinomas and neuroendocrine tumours.

57. D Koilocytosis

Cervical intraepithelial neoplasia (CIN) is a premalignant condition that if left untreated has the potential to become cervical cancer. CIN is divided into three grades depending on the epithelial depth of the dysplastic changes occurring in the cells of the transformation zone of the cervix. CIN is caused by chronic human papillomavirus infection, predominantly virus types 16 and 18. Liquid cytology now provides the method used for screening for CIN in the UK.

Cytological changes characteristic of CIN of dysplasia include poikilocytosis (abnormally shaped cells), an increased nuclear:cytoplasmic ratio, nuclear hyperchromasia, multinucleated cells and evidence of increased mitoses, suggesting a high cell turnover.

Koilocytosis refers to presence of cells infected with HPV, which have abnormally large and irregularly shaped nuclei. See **Table 16.5** for classification of CIN.

Table 16.5 Histology, management and malignant potential of cervical intraepithelial neoplasia (CIN)

Grade	Thickness of squamous epithelium affected	Current monitoring and treatment	Malignant potential
CIN I	Basal 1/3	Conservative: 6 monthly colposcopy and repeat cytology LLETZ	Low malignant potential (around 1%); spontaneous regression common
CIN II	Basal 2/3	LLETZ treatment required	Approx. 5% in 10 years
CIN III	> 2/3 to full thickness affected	LLETZ treatment required	20–30% in 10 years

LLETZ, large loop excision of transformation zone.

58. C Colliquative necrosis

Necrosis describes the death of living cells following an insult. It is associated with cell shrinkage, and the breakdown of cellular contents. During necrosis there is pyknosis, karyolysis and karyorrhexis of the nucleus and its contents and enzymatic degradation with the release of inflammatory mediators. The form of necrosis that occurs is secondary to the form of insult and the tissues involved. In cerebral infarction there is colliquative necrosis whereby enzymatic degradation of cellular material may lead to affected tissue turning into a fluid form. Myocardial infarction typifies coagulative necrosis caused by hypoxic damage. Caseous necrosis is seen in tuberculosis where foci of infected necrotic tissue have a soft cheese-like appearance. Fat necrosis occurs in and around peritoneal tissue; it is associated with pancreatic damage and breast tissue whereby trauma to adipocytes leads to an inflammatory reaction with subsequent scarring and sometimes with calcium deposition leading to calcium soap formation. Gangrenous necrosis is not a distinct form of necrosis; however, it describes the appearance of black, dead tissue. Gangrene usually occurs in the absence of an adequate blood supply. Gangrene can be described as dry (for example, in an ischaemic limb), wet (for example, in the presence of Gram-negative bacterial infection), and finally as gas gangrene (in the presence of gas-producing bacteria such as *Clostridium perfringens*).

59. E Protein C deficiency

Thrombophilia may be inherited or acquired. These hypercoagulable states all increase the risk of thrombus formation. Protein C deficiency is an autosomal dominant condition. Protein C acts against activated factor V and VIII, which are coagulation factors, as well as augmenting fibrinolysis. Hence, in the presence of protein C deficiency there is an increased risk of venous thrombosis. Other inherited thrombophilias include factor V Leiden, protein S deficiency, anti-thrombin deficiency and hyperhomocystinaemia.

60. A Antiphospholipid syndrome

Antiphospholipid syndrome is an acquired thrombophilia associated with increased risk of thrombosis, recurrent miscarriage, stillbirth and pre-eclampsia in the presence of persistent antiphospholipid antibodies such as anticardiolipin antibodies and lupus anticoagulant. Other forms of acquired thrombophilia include heparin-induced thrombocytopaenia (HIT) and paroxysmal nocturnal haemoglobinuria. HIT occurs when administration of heparin and subsequent binding to platelets leads to antibody production, which subsequently causes platelet activation and subsequent thrombosis. Paroxysmal nocturnal haemoglobinuria is a rare disorder of bone marrow associated with anaemia and thrombosis. Antithrombin III deficiency, dysfibrinogenemia, factor V Leiden and protein S are all inherited thrombophilias.

61. C 10 mSV

The unit of measurement for effective radiation dose is Sieverts. The background radiation is approximately 3 mSv per year.

Below is a table of some common imaging modalities and their approximate radiation dose:

Imaging modality	Effective radiation dose (mSV)
Chest radiograph	0.1
Chest CT	7
CT of the abdomen or pelvis	10
DEXA scan	0.001
Mammogram	0.4

62. B Modulated Blend 1 mode

Cutting mode of diathermy involves continuous waveform, whereas coagulation mode involves intermittent waveform.

There are three different types of modulated electrosurgery modes. Blend 1 involves 50% with current on and 50% with current off. Blend 2 involves 40% on and 60% off, whilst Blend 3 involves 25% on and 75% off.

63. C 78

Radioisotopes are radioactive isotopes of different elements. The same element can have different isotopes with the same number of protons but differing numbers of neutrons. The isotopes are represented using the following method:

A = Mass number = protons + neutrons

X = Chemical symbol of element

Z = Atomic number = proton

64. A Epithelial surface damage

Radiotherapy is used in the treatment of a wide range of malignancies; patients exposed to it may experience a number of side effects, both early and late. Epithelial surface damage is an example of an acute side effect of radiotherapy and may manifest in the form of mouth ulcers. Radiotherapy for vulval cancer is particularly associated with severe skin reactions, due to the high dosages of radiation required. Other acute side effects of radiotherapy include gastrointestinal symptoms, cystitis, fatigue and oedema. **Table 16.6** lists acute and late side effects of radiotherapy.

Table 16.6 Side-effects of radiotherapy	
Acute	**Late**
• Oedema	• Lymphoedema
• Gastrointestinal symptoms: nausea, vomiting, diarrhoea, abdominal pain	• Hair loss
	• Development of further cancers
• Fatigue	• Tissue fibrosis
• Epithelial surface damage, e.g. mouth ulcers	• Infertility

65. A Immediately after delivery of the placenta

Provision of advice and access to contraception is often neglected in the period immediately after a baby is born. However, it is possible to avoid unwanted pregnancies in the postpartum period through the immediate provision of contraception if the patient wants. Ideally a woman's intentions for contraception should have been discussed in the antenatal setting, with further information and access to contraception available during admission for delivery, and once again at any postnatal reviews. An intrauterine device (IUD) is a highly effective form of contraception that can be inserted immediately after the delivery of the placenta, up until 48 hours post-delivery (it can also be fitted during caesarean section). If the IUD is not inserted in this immediate period then insertion should be delayed until six weeks post-partum, because of the risk of perforating the post-partum uterus.

66. A Admit for intravenous antibiotics and supportive care

Pelvic inflammatory disease (PID) is a common problem in young women. Untreated PID can lead to long-term subfertility, be associated with chronic pelvic pain and increases the risk of ectopic pregnancy. Hence, a low threshold for treatment is required. Admission to hospital may be necessary in clinically severe cases, and when other surgical emergencies need to be excluded. Intravenous antibiotics for at least 24 hours are recommended. Women should be given a detailed explanation of the diagnosis and its possible long-term implications, and the importance of contact tracing should be reinforced.

67. B She is immune to chickenpox and no further action needs to be taken

The incubation period of chickenpox is 1–3 weeks. Chickenpox is infectious from 48 hours before the rash appears and remains so until the vesicles crust over. If a woman is not immune, varicella vaccination can be offered pre-pregnancy or postpartum. Women who are varicella zoster virus IgG-negative should avoid contact with chickenpox and shingles in pregnancy. Varicella zoster immunoglobulin (VZIG) should be given to non-immune pregnant women who have been exposed. VZIG should not be given once chickenpox has developed. Chickenpox in the first trimester does not increase risk of miscarriage.

68. E Polycystic ovarian syndrome

Polycystic ovarian syndrome is one of the most common endocrine conditions associated with subfertility and anovulation. The hormone picture is usually 1:3 ratio of early follicular phase follicle-stimulating hormone (FSH):luteinising hormone (LH) along with an ovulatory day 21 progesterone (<30 ng/mL) levels. Women with premature menopause will also have raised FSH and LH levels in the early follicular phase. Endometriosis and Asherman's syndrome do not alter the FSH/LH ratio. Hypogonadotrophic hypogonadism results in very low FSH and LH levels without alteration to the ratio.

69. A A repeat sample should be performed in 30 minutes

This fetal blood sample (FBS) shows a pH of 7.24, which is classified as suspicious. The sample should be repeated in no more than 30 minutes, or sooner if clinically indicated. See **Table 16.7** for a FBS action plan.

Table 16.7 Interpretation of fetal blood sampling (FBS) results		
Result (pH)	**Interpretation**	**Action**
≥7.25	Normal	Repeat FBS if cardiotocograph remains pathological or suspicious
7.21–7.24	Suspicious	Repeat FBS in 30 minutes or sooner if indicated
≤7.20	Abnormal	Delivery

70. E Send urine for microscopy and culture and treat if positive

Urine tract infection (UTI) is defined as the presence of 100,000/mL organisms in an asymptomatic patient or 100/mL organisms with increased white cell count in a symptomatic patient. In an asymptomatic patient, the diagnosis of a urinary tract infection should be made once the presence of a pathogen has been confirmed on culture. Asymptomatic bacteriuria is the presence of 100,000/mL of organisms in the absence of symptoms on at least two occasions. These are treated, as there is a risk of cystitis and ascending infection, which may increase maternal or fetal morbidity.

Urinalysis should be performed on pregnant women routinely at all antenatal clinic visits. The presence of protein, leucocytes and nitrites all suggest the presence of a UTI. A renal ultrasound scan would only be indicated in the presence of recurrent pyelonephritis or if renal abnormality or disease is suspected.

71. E Sickle cell trait

Sickle cell conditions are due to the production of abnormal β peptide chains leading to abnormal haemoglobin. The gene that codes for the β chain of haemoglobin has an amino acid substitution, which results in the production of HbS rather than HbA. Individuals with sickle cell anaemia are homozygous with HbSS. Heterozygotes have HbAS and have sickle cell trait. Sickle cell trait is thought to be protective against *Plasmodium falciparum* malaria. Sickle cell anaemia results in the production of fragile erythrocytes, which leads to their early destruction and subsequent haemolysis. Ideally these patients should have pre-pregnancy counselling and their partner should be screened. If this has not been undertaken prior to conception, then it should be arranged as soon as it is identified to determine the risk of HbSS in the fetus. In sickle cell trait there may be mild anaemia, however there is usually no evidence of haemolysis, i.e. normal lactate dehydrogenase, bilirubin and a normal reticulocyte count.

72. D 110–160 beats per minute

Cardiotocography (CTG) or electronic fetal monitoring is commonly used during pregnancy and labour to determine fetal wellbeing. Different parameters are studied including baseline fetal heart rate, which is considered normal if between 110–160 beats per minute. Fetal cardiac activity is controlled via the sympathetic and parasympathetic autonomic nervous systems, with other influences coming from oxygenation and baroreceptors. Fetal baseline heart rate generally falls as the pregnancy increases and this is a result of the parasympathetic system becoming more developed. Intrapartum fetal tachycardia, when associated with maternal tachycardia, may be as a result of infection, and chorioamnionitis should be considered.

73. E Varicella zoster – previous exposure

Varicella zoster virus is a member of the herpes virus family and causes chickenpox. The majority of adults in the UK are immune to chickenpox. It is transmitted via droplet infection and has a relatively long incubation period of approximately 2 weeks. Chickenpox infection is more severe in pregnancy and there is a higher rate of complications, such as varicella pneumonitis. Once there has been exposure to the virus there will be initial production of varicella IgM antibodies, followed by the production of long-term immunity through IgG antibodies. In the case illustrated, the patient has IgG positive result and is therefore immune to varicella zoster through previous exposure. There is therefore no risk to the fetus and no indication for immunoglobulin. If IgM was positive and IgG negative, this would suggest recent infection with no prior immunity and this would be an indication for immunoglobulin.

74. C > 0.3 g

Urinary protein excretion of >0.3 g in 24 hours indicates a significant level of proteinuria. This may be found in conditions such as pre-eclampsia or pre-existing renal disease. Severe proteinuria may not always be associated with significantly raised blood pressure and may be due to long-standing renal damage and should be investigated.

75. D Type II

Rhesus (Rh) D antigen is carried on erythrocytes. If a child is born to an Rh-negative mother and the father is Rh positive, he or she may express Rh D on their erythrocytes. If fetal erythrocytes pass into the maternal circulation or if Rh D positive blood is transfused into the mother, then sensitisation may occur; the mother will produce antibodies. In subsequent pregnancies, fetal erythrocytes may cross the placenta and stimulate a memory response, leading to the production of IgG antibodies, which destroy fetal erythrocytes. Anti-D immunoprophylaxis, using anti-D immunoglobulin, during pregnancy and in the immediate postnatal period prevents the development of maternal anti-D antibodies.

76. D

| Monomer | Only immunoglobulin to cross the placenta |

Immunoglobulins, also known as antibodies, are formed by B cells. There are five different classes of human immunoglobulin, which differ in both their structure and function. Immunoglobin (IgG) is the predominant immunoglobulin found in serum and is the only form of immunoglobulin that is able to cross the placenta and therefore results in immunity in the fetus. It is also the longest living antibody class, with a half-life of around 3 weeks. There are four IgG subclasses. Named IgG 1–4, this class of immunoglobulin is the predominant form involved in the secondary immune response. IgG antibodies are good at fixing complement, as well as opsonising targets, such as bacteria, for phagocytosis by cells such as macrophages.

77. B Cleavage of C3 into C3a and C3b

The complement system consists of around 20 proteins, which are produced in a cascade and aim to attack pathogens. Although the complement cascade forms part of the innate immune system, it can also be activated by the adaptive immune system. Traditionally the complement cascade is described as being activated by three different pathways. The classical complement pathway occurs in response to activation of the complement protein C1 to antigen-antibody complexes. The alternative activation pathway does not rely on the presence of activated antibody complexes and instead starts with the activation of the complement protein C3. The third activation pathway is the lectin activation pathway. The liver produces mannose-binding lectin. It forms a complex with a further protein called MASP. When the lectin binds to a pathogen containing mannose, the MASP protein converts the C3 complement protein to C3b and the cascade begins. Despite three different activation pathways, the common step in all is the cleavage of the complement protein C3 to C3a and C3b (**Figure 16.2**).

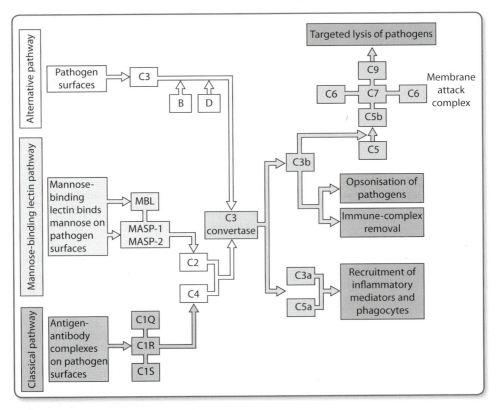

Figure 16.2 Complement activation pathways.

78. B Haemostasis

After an insult, the processes involved in acute inflammation are aimed at removing the source of the trauma and encouraging healing. Acute inflammation is associated with a series of vascular changes, which aim to bring key components of the inflammatory response to the site of injury. Vasodilation occurs rapidly after an insult in response to mediators such as histamine. This leads to increased blood flow to the traumatised area, with associated hyperaemia. Vascular permeability also increases, allowing the passage of proteins, leucocytes and fluid from the vasculature into the surrounding tissues. The movement of protein-rich fluid out of the vasculature is associated with increased hydrostatic pressure. With a reduction in intravascular volume there is an element of haemostasis, also contributing to local hyperaemia.

Both fibroblast infiltration and a high concentration of monocytes are typical of chronic inflammation rather than acute.

79. A *Actinomyces israelii*

The Gram-positive bacteria *Actinomyces israelii* is a commensal of the colon, mouth and vagina. It is the commonest cause of actinomycosis, a chronic, suppurative and granulomatous inflammatory infection. The majority of cases of actinomycosis affect the cervicofacial area, classically presenting as painless facial lumps; however, thoracic, abdominal and pelvic forms do occasionally occur. Diagnosis of pelvic actinomycosis is usually made from histological samples taken during surgery and has been associated with intrauterine contraceptive devices which have been in situ for long periods of time. The presence of sulphur granules is characteristic of actinomyces infection.

80. C *Chlamydia trachomatis*

The boyfriend's symptoms are suggestive of a urethritis, which from the list of given options, the cause is most likely to be Chlamydia infection. It is caused by *Chlamydia trachomatis*, a Gram-negative intracellular bacterium, which infects squamocolumnar epithelial cells. Chlamydia infection is often asymptomatic, especially in women. Women may notice postcoital or intermenstrual bleeding, dysuria and low abdominal pain, whereas men may experience dysuria, penile discharge and scrotal pain. Chlamydia infection is the commonest cause of pelvic inflammatory disease and may go on to cause subfertility and increased risk of ectopic pregnancy. Treatment regimens for uncomplicated Chlamydial infection include azithromycin, doxycycline and erythromycin.

81. D *Treponema pallidum pallidum*

Syphilis is caused by the spirochete *Treponema pallidum pallidum*. Primary syphilis typically presents with a painless genital ulcer (a chancre) alongside inguinal lymphadenopathy, occurring 10–90 days after infection. Secondary syphilis develops within 2 years of infection and tertiary syphilis after this period. Screening tests for syphilis include the venereal disease research laboratory (VDRL) carbon antigen test and the rapid plasma regain test, both of which can give false positives. More specific tests for syphilis include fluorescent treponema antibody absorption test; however, these tests can give a positive result when there is infection from other treponema, such as the causative agents of yaw, bejel and pinta. Syphilis in pregnancy is associated with stillbirth, preterm delivery and congenital defects.

82. B *Clostridium perfringens*

Gas gangrene is most commonly caused by *Clostridium perfringens*; however, it can also be caused by other species of anaerobic bacteria including *Clostridium septicum*, *Klebsiella pneumoniae* and *Escherichia coli*. Exotoxins produced by the bacteria lead to necrotic tissue damage and sepsis often requiring amputation of the affected tissue. Gas gangrene was historically associated with war injuries, where open wounds were exposed to these soil-loving bacterium. Today, risk factors for the development of gas gangrene include trauma such as open fractures and burns, alongside malignancy of the gastrointestinal tract, diabetes mellitus, chronic alcohol abuse and as a rare post-surgical complication.

83. B *Escherichia coli*

Uncomplicated urinary tract infections (UTIs) are common in women, particularly during pregnancy. The most common causative organism of uncomplicated urinary tract infection is *Escherichia coli*, a gastrointestinal commensal. Suitable antibiotics for the treatment of a proven *E. coli* UTI in pregnancy include cefalexin and nitrofurantoin (should be avoided at term due to risk of neonatal haemolysis). *Klebsiella pneumoniae*, *Proteus mirabilis* and *Citrobacter freundii* are also Gram-negative commensals of the gastrointestinal tract and therefore may all cause infection of the urinary tract, particularly in women due to the close proximity of the anus and the urethra.

Staphylococcus saprophyticus is a common cause of urinary tract infection in sexually active women.

84. C Human herpesvirus 8

Kaposi's sarcoma is caused by human herpesvirus 8; although not always coexistent with HIV infection, Kaposi's sarcoma is considered an AIDS-defining illness, whereby reduced immune-surveillance can result in its characteristic lesions of the skin, respiratory and gastrointestinal tract. Human herpesvirus 4, more commonly known as Epstein–Barr virus, is the causative agent of infectious mononucleosis; it is also associated with several forms of lymphoproliferative neoplasias, e.g. Burkitt's lymphoma, nasopharyngeal carcinoma and Hodgkin's lymphoma.

85. D Recent infection with parvovirus B19

Both parvovirus 19 and rubella infection may present with a rash. If contracted in pregnancy both viruses have implications for the fetus, and therefore rapidly establishing the immune status of the mother is vital, as this will guide the further management of the pregnancy. It is important to send urgent serology requesting specific IgG and IgM status for each virus. The presence of IgG suggests previous exposure to an antigen, whether in the form of a vaccine or through contracting the virus. Development of IgM is an acute event and occurs after exposure to the antigen. In this patient, the serology results for rubella suggests either previous exposure or immunisation to rubella, without any evidence of acute infection.

Specific parvovirus B19 serology indicated recent infection with parvovirus B19. Parvovirus B19 has been implicated with pregnancy loss and with fetal hydrops and anaemia.

86. B Chorioamnionitis

The risk of vertical transmission of HIV is highest at delivery. In non-breastfeeding untreated European women vertical transmission of HIV occurs in around 20% of cases. Use of highly active anti-retroviral therapy (HAART) has reduced vertical transmission in treated women to < 2%. Nevertheless, the management of the delivery and postnatal period requires planning and a multidisciplinary team approach. Prematurity, chorioamnionitis, prolonged rupture of membranes and breastfeeding all increase the risk of transmission. Elective caesarean section is the recommended mode of delivery for certain cases, i.e. HIV positive women not using HAART, women with a viral load above 50 copies/mL or if there is coexistent hepatitis C. A planned vaginal delivery may be suitable for women with viral loads < 50 copies/mL who are using HAART.

87. D Submucosal

Uterine fibroids, also known as leiomyomas, are benign growths of smooth muscle, which arise from the myometrium of the uterus. They can be classified according to their location. Women with fibroids may complain of menorrhagia, dysmenorrhoea, and problems with urinary frequency and hesitancy. In severe cases fibroids may be associated with anaemia and urinary retention. Reduced fertility may also be associated with fibroids depending on their size and location. Fibroids are more common in women of Afro-Caribbean origin and in obese women. Treatment options include hormone therapy such as GnRH analogues to cause pre-operative shrinkage, myomectomy, uterine artery embolisation and hysterectomy. Rarely fibroids may undergo malignant change and become leiomyosarcomas (**Figure 16.3**).

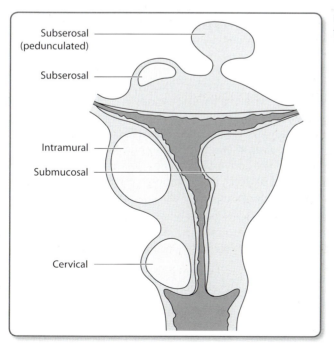

Subserosal (pedunculated)

Subserosal

Intramural

Submucosal

Cervical

Figure 16.3 Location of uterine fibroids.

88. D Mesenchyme

Sarcomas are malignant tumours of connective tissues i.e. bone, muscle and cartilage. These mesenchymal tumours form from tissue that was originally embryonic mesoderm. They are highly vascular tumours, which grow quickly and can metastasise via the bloodstream to the lungs and other sites. On microscopy they consist of spindle cells. Sarcomas may be treated using radiotherapy, chemotherapy or surgical excision.

The commonest forms of sarcomas are gastrointestinal stromal image (GIST). Other examples of sarcomas include osteosarcoma, Botryoides sarcoma, malignant schwannoma and chondrosarcoma. Low grade tumours may be effectively surgically excised, however higher grade forms may respond to both radiotherapy and chemotherapy.

89. B Hyperparathyroidism

Osteoporosis is a condition associated with significantly reduced bone density. Osteoporosis is more common in women and affects large numbers after the menopause. Risk factors for osteoporosis include: having a low BMI, smoking, calcium deficiency, excess alcohol intake, minimal exercise, family history and corticosteroid usage. Osteoporosis is also common in states of hypogonadism, for example in individuals with Kallman syndrome. Prevention of osteoporosis is possible by early recognition of modifiable risk factors such as smoking and low levels of weight-bearing exercise. Individuals with osteoporosis may benefit from the usage of biphosphonates and calcium supplementation.

90. E Transformation from one type of differentiated cell to another type of cell

Metaplasia represents the benign change from one form of differentiated type of cell to another type of differentiated cell. Metaplasia typically occurs in response to an irritant stimulus, whereby the cell type of a tissue changes in order to cope with the stresses of the irritant (**Figure 16.4**). This change in cell phenotype may be reversible, especially when the 'stressful stimulus' is removed. Examples of metaplastic change include the change from columnar epithelium to squamous epithelium in the transition zone of the cervix, and the conversion of the squamous epithelium to transitional epithelium in cases of Barrett's oesophagus, which occur due to chronic acid exposure. Although metaplastic change in itself is benign, persistent exposure to irritants may eventually lead to dysplasia and potentially neoplastic change.

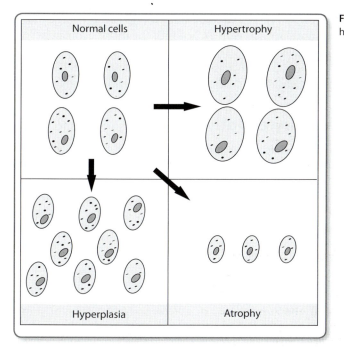

Figure 16.4 Hypertrophy, hyperplasia and atrophy.

---

91. A Basophils

Histamine (5-hydroxytryptamine) is a significant contributor to the immediate response in acute inflammation and is a vasoactive amine. It is predominantly produced by local mast cells, but also by basophils and platelets. Histamine is typically stored in mast cell granules and released during a process called degranulation following mast cell activation. This activation may occur in response to stimuli, such as mast cell antibody binding, following complement activation and in direct response to injury. The main action of histamine is vascular dilatation, but it is also involved in increasing vascular permeability.

---

92. D 48–92 hours

The process of cutaneous wound healing occurs with initial inflammation, followed by proliferation and then maturation. Healing by primary intention follows surgical incision closed by suturing. The initial surgical incision causes platelets to rapidly gather to form a clot, which instigates the inflammatory response. Healing by secondary intention occurs when there is a traumatic wound causing large loss of cells and tissues. Neutrophils appear with 24 hours of the insult. Fibroblasts proliferate in the first 24–72 hours forming granulation tissue, which fills the wound within 1 week. Neutrophils are replaced by macrophages within 48–96 hours. Leucocyte infiltration and increased vascularity is present for up to 14 days.

93. B Glomerular capillary endotheliosis

Pre-eclampsia is a complex condition that affects many body systems, including the kidneys, and affects both function and morphology. It leads to the glomerulus becoming hypertrophied with reduced perfusion as a result of hypertrophy of intracapillary cells. The reactive changes of the kidney are described as glomerular capillary endotheliosis. The extent to which the kidneys are affected varies according to the location of the lesion but in severe cases may involve the whole of the renal cortex.

94. A Increase in the number of cells

Hyperplasia is an increase in the number of cells as a response to a specific stimulus. Hypertrophy is an increase in the size of the cells. Hyperplasia is often benign, as in benign prostatic hyperplasia, but can sometimes manifest as a premalignant condition. The microscopic and macroscopic appearance of the cells remains the same, but there are an increased number of them present. Other examples of cellular hyperplasia include the growth of glandular breast tissue during pregnancy, endometrial hyperplasia and the hyperplasia of the adrenal cortex seen in Cushing's disease (**Figure 16.4**).

95. C Dopamine receptor D2 agonist

Prolactin is under inhibitory control by dopamine. In cases of stillbirth, woman should be advised that dopamine agonists successfully suppress lactation in the large majority, and are well tolerated. Cabergoline has been demonstrated to be superior to Bromocriptine in terms of ease of use and adverse effects. Dopamine agonists are contra-indicated in women with hypertension and pre-eclampsia.

96. A Labetolol

The guidelines on hypertension in pregnancy depend on severity. **Table 16.8** summarises the different management strategies advised. Any degree of hypertension in pregnancy requires hospital admission in the first instance to control the blood pressure. The target diastolic blood pressure should be between 80-100 mmHg, with a target systolic blood pressure of less than 150 mmHg.

Table 16.8 Initial treatment of hypertension in pregnancy

	Blood pressure (mmHg)	Treatment required	Frequency of blood pressure checks
Mild	140/90 – 149/99	Observation	At least QDS
Moderate	150/100 – 159/109	Oral labetolol as first line	At least QDS
Severe	160/110 or higher	Oral labetolol as first line	More than QDS, as clinically indicated

97. C Ergometrine

The causes of postpartum haemorrhage can be categorised into four, summarised as the "four T's": Tone, Trauma, Tissue, and Thrombin.

Prophylactic oxytocics have been shown to reduce the risk of postpartum haemorrhage by about 60%.

Syntometrine is a combined agent containing oxytocin and ergometrine. Syntometrine may be used in the absence of hypertension. Ergometrine is an ergot alkaloid, whereas misoprostol is a prostaglandin E1 analogue.

98. A Anti-progesterone

A combination of mifepristone and a prostaglandin is considered the first line intervention for induction of labour in late intrauterine fetal death. Mifepristone is an anti-progesterone, and helps to soften and dilate the cervix, thus priming for prostaglandin administration.

99. E Inhibits folic acid metabolism

Medical management (with methotrexate) should be offered if:

- Women are able to attend appropriate follow up, and
- Have no significant pain, and
- Ultrasound scan confirms an unruptured ectopic smaller than 35mm, and
- No visible heartbeat with no intrauterine pregnancy, and
- A β-HCG level less than 1500 IU/litre.

Surgical management should be offered as first line to women who are unable to attend appropriate follow-up, or have significant pain, an ultrasound confirming an adnexal mass measuring 35 mm or larger, or a visible heartbeat, or if b-HCG is more than 5000 IU/litre.

100. C 10 days LMWH

Any woman with two current risk factors should be considered for prophylactic low molecular weight heparin (LMWH) for 10 days postpartum. Risk factors include age > 35 years, BMI more than or equal to $30\,kg/m^2$, parity more than or equal to 3, smoking, multiple pregnancy, pre-eclampsia, caesarean section, prolonged labour and postpartum haemorrhage.

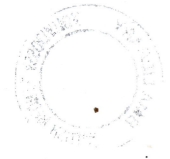